The Gospel of Longevity

By
JAMES R. STROLE
with JOSEPH BARDIN

The Gospel of Longevity

For permission requests, write to the publisher, addressed "Attention: Permissions Coordinator" reception@markvictorhansen.com

Quantity sales special discounts are available on quantity purchases by corporations, associations, and others. For details, contact the publisher at reception@markvictorhansen.com

Orders by U.S. trade bookstores and wholesalers.
Email: reception@markvictorhansen.com

Manufactured and printed in the United States of America distributed globally by markvictorhansenlibrary.com

New York | Los Angeles | London | Sydney

ISBN: 979-8-88581-243-6 Hardback
ISBN: 979-8-88581-244-3 Paperback
ISBN: 979-8-88581-245-0 eBook

Table of Contents

Testimonials

"A soul-stirring perspective that brings together science and spirituality for everyone excited about the singularity and longevity escape velocity. It covers the crucial issue that we will need to know how to navigate the enormous intellect we will have when we merge artificial intelligence with our biological mind."

— Ray Kurzweil, futurist, inventor and author

"God wants you to live long, prosper, and be in good health. This book will tell you how to stop striving for it and start thriving with it."

— Rev. Eula M. Dent Eikerenkoetter, "Mrs. Rev. Ike"

"In The Gospel of Longevity Strole displays his courage and passion with relentless honesty on how he came to be the longevity leader he is today."

— Dr. Aubrey de Grey, President and
Chief Science Officer of LEV Foundation

"Longevity and immortality are central to Judaism as a physical reality in this world. Strole makes this vision personal for our time with spirit and dedication."

— Rabbi Or Shraga, Vetek Association

"James Strole brings together the spiritual and the scientific to give us a view of immortality that is truly inspirational and available right now."

— Ed Jones, Academy Award winning producer

"Life driven by survival slowly diminishes the soul and distances us from the peace God intends for us. This book is a powerful reminder that true longevity flows from spiritual renewal and a life anchored in grace—one marked by trust and joy rather than fear and striving."

— Daniel Rodas, certified Chaplain, Apostle, Signs and Wonders International Ministries

"I can't see us radically extending life without adopting the outlook James presents in this book. And really, what would be the point?"

— Dr. Bill Andrews, Sierra Sciences, groundbreaking longevity scientist

Dedication

To my late partner Bernadeane who was a guiding light to me and many around her and was an inspiration for this book and for my continued exploration of the spirit of immortality, which shone so brightly in her.

* * * *

To Charles Paul Brown, a visionary leader in his own right, and one of the first to openly express that physical immortality is possible, who was a great inspiration to both Bernie and me.

* * * *

To my mother, Eunice Strole, who encouraged me from a young age to seek the deeper truths in life, treat my body as sacred, and to never stop on myself.

* * * *

And to all the scientists and activists working to cure aging so that we can experience our full humanity.

Prologue

I wrote this book to show people there's a way out of the survival anxiety that is killing all of us. Working over four decades in longevity, I've looked at everything that ages us. And there are many factors. But nothing breaks us down physically, nothing stunts our emotional and spiritual growth like the pressure and drive of living within the system of survival.

The problem is we've lived this way so long, we think it's normal. We think it's the only way. But it's not the only way, and that's what I'm going to show you in this book. You can get out from under the burdens of survival and the results are miraculous.

I know because about four years ago I had an experience that changed me, and consequently altered my entire way of life. And I'm so grateful for this. It's not an exaggeration to say I was reborn. I took on a new way of thinking, a new way of feeling, and a new way of being. Without the trauma of survival. And in this book, you'll learn how this change happened to me.

When people hear about change, they tend to think it has to be tough. The bigger the change, the bigger the struggle. No pain, no gain and all that. But this transformation has been entirely without pain. It's been nothing but joy and creation and that continues to this day.

That's why I want to share it with you. Because if we're going to live our full potential for longevity, we need a strength and faith and joy that is sustainable. Not just for today, but for the long term. And that's what this book is about.

CHAPTER 1

Be Reborn: A New Witnessing of Life

"Ask, and it shall be given you; seek, and ye shall find; knock, and it shall be opened unto you."

— Matthew 7:7

I was feeling this deep longing for two or three weeks and I couldn't get away from it. During the day, I was busy with work, but as soon as I got quiet, when I lay down to go to sleep, there it was—this pressure building in me from within. So much so, that one night before bed, I just wanted a break from it all.

I took out my iPad to see what I could find to get my mind off all the seriousness. I turned on Netflix to look for something interesting to watch. I clicked through movies and documentaries, but nothing caught my eye. I guess I was also tired of the same old same old on TV.

The funny thing is when you're undergoing real travail, or deep soul reflection, you can't get away from it. You might think you are, but even what you do to try to escape, ends up bringing you right back to what you're trying to get away from. I don't really know why it caught my eye, but I stopped on a series called *The Chosen*, about the life of Jesus.

Yes, this is about an experience with Jesus. No, I am not religious. I am an immortalist who believes that we should all have the opportunity to live as long as we wish. In my case, I would certainly choose to live indefinitely. I think everyone would choose this if they believed it was possible and were feeling good enough, but that's still a personal choice.

How are we going to get there? I believe that science and technology are advancing fast enough to make this possible in our lifetimes, but it's going to take a big push from people who aren't afraid to step out of the mortality paradigm. I like to cite my friend, Ray Kurzweil, the great inventor and futurist, who has predicted we'll reach longevity escape velocity by 2030, which is right around the corner.

To be clear, I'm talking about physical immortality, not spiritual immortality. I'm talking about the combination of science and the power of human intention to create a new paradigm in human living. What does all this have to do with Jesus? That is the focus of this book.

I was born into Christianity but by the time I was ten years old, my had mother had left the Presbyterian Church, saying "the word was dead." She took me to hear all kinds of speakers and ministers and anyone who had some kind of enlightenment to share. I did programs such as Psycho-Cybernetics, which inspired people like Tony Robbins, and I studied yoga.

I admired Jesus, the man. I'd always loved stories about Jesus—how he cared about all people, the great expressions of life and passion he gave, such as the Sermon on the Mount, and his power to heal people and impact them for the better. But I didn't think I had much more to learn from him. I was working on immortality, and he had died, so how much could I take from his life, which as we all know, ended in death—probably the most famous death in history.

Still, something made me stop and consider this show. The series was well reviewed and I saw that it was crowdfunded and wasn't connected to any specific denomination or faith. I got interested and thought I would give it a try.

The show was well done—the cinematography, the writing all struck me as being good quality. It started with scenes showing life in ancient Israel, which seemed realistic, but didn't exactly grab me. I'd been to Israel numerous times to speak on immortality, so I was familiar with a lot of the history. The character of Jesus doesn't appear until the final scene of the first episode when he releases Mary Magdalene from the demons that torment her.

My Quickening

I watched as Jesus freed Mary Magdalene from her trauma simply by calling her name. He says: "I have called you by name, you are mine." It turns out that this is a direct quote from the prophet Isaiah, showing that Jesus was drawing from a long line of inspiration, but more about that in Chapter 3.

I watched the show as Jesus changed the chemistry in Mary Magdalene's body from that of a tortured person traumatized by terrible experiences and by her own sense of shame, all of which threatened to drive her out of her mind, into a person that was bright, stable, and suddenly at peace.

As I watched the story of Jesus healing Mary Magdalene, something happened to me.

I knew I was watching an actor, named Jonathan Roumie, and that he was performing lines from a script written for the show, many of which are taken directly from the New Testament. But everything the character of Jesus said seemed to penetrate into me. I didn't know what was going on but I knew it felt good. I had wanted to feel something fresh, and this was definitely that.

As an immortalist, I've always felt that being open to the unknown is essential. When we think we know everything, we're dead already. This is true of scientific innovation, where we have to be ready to pivot away from assumptions when they prove to be no longer valid, even those that have been institutionally accepted. The same is true of our own personal experience. Who we think we are, and how we think we are supposed to move can't be fixed. We also need to explore what is new and unfamiliar within our own selves.

I was open to allowing this new experience to happen inside me. As I was watching the story of Mary Magdalene unfold, I felt like my own name had been called. I didn't know what or why or how, but I was witnessing something very powerful in my own body. I felt light, like my own burdens had been lifted, at least for the moment.

I slept well that night and I figured that would be that. I love inspirational movies and music, but you don't expect the uplift that comes from them to take you to a new level of living. The inspiration hits you, and you enjoy it, until it's gone and you're back in real life.

But the next morning, I was still feeling good. I had been waking up heavy every morning since this travail had started, which wasn't like me, but was starting to be normal. I expected to feel the same way, but instead, when I got up, I was excited and a lightness permeated my body. I thought, great, maybe this relief from my heaviness will last a couple days instead of just one.

The Lifting of the Veil

If ever there was a case for binge-watching a streaming show, this was it. Whatever was happening to me, I wanted more of it, and since this show was the stimulus, I went back for more. As I watched the following episodes of the show and the ministry of Jesus took form, the feeling of peace and clarity that had come to me the night before didn't dim at all, if anything it became stronger. It was as if a veil started to lift, and I was able to see things that had been obscured to me before.

As I'm writing this, I realize how charged a topic Jesus is for many people. I don't begrudge anyone reading this book having a reaction for or against, because I know how programmed we all are on the topic. Everyone seems to have an opinion about Jesus. That in itself is remarkable and suggests that there was something very special and potent about him that enabled him to make such a broad impact that lasts until today.

Even the staunchest atheist knows who Jesus is, and probably has an opinion about him. Unfortunately, the meaning of the life of Jesus has been hijacked by religion. Whatever it is that bothers people about Jesus is almost always because of this. It's not Jesus that pushes their buttons; it's the religious training they received at some point in their life in the name of Jesus.

The question is what exactly was the impact Jesus made? Non-Christians tend to view him as a social activist who advocated for greater justice in the world. While this is true, it also leaves out a lot, including the miracles he's reported to have performed. Also, just being someone who speaks for social justice doesn't account for the depth of feeling people hold for him.

Biblical prophets like Isaiah, Amos, Micah, and others called for justice and compassion. Socrates tried to teach ethics and justice in ancient Greece. Mary Wollstonecraft was an early feminist in England in the 1700s. Frederick Douglass spoke for the abolition of slavery in the US. Voltaire advocated against authoritarianism during the French Enlightenment. History remembers these people, but none are beloved on a personal level like Jesus is.

Christians emphasize the miracles of Jesus as evidence of his divinity, but then tend to make him perfect, and therefore, not a human being whose passion and inspiration we can aspire to embody. Also, they see his worth in the sacrifice of his life, supposedly to cleanse the sins of humanity. How someone dying accomplishes this is not at all clear, at least not to me. Even the notion of wanting someone else to die for your sins so you can live seems to create as much trouble as it solves, if not more. It means death for one, and guilt for the other. And what kind of God would require that sort of payment? Clearly, not the God of benevolence and justice that Christianity describes.

As I watched the famous story of Jesus whipping the money changers out of the temple compound, I saw it wasn't the commerce that offended him, it was the primitiveness of sacrifice. The irony that religion seeks to find meaning in Jesus as a sacrificial lamb makes his death what matters and misses the real message, which was his life.

Sacrifice to appease angry, threatening gods is hardly a new concept. Archeological evidence of ritual burials and offerings goes back to Paleolithic and Neolithic times. This is important because Jesus is considered a revolutionary figure, especially by those who claim to love him. But what was the change he was seeking to bring? The idea that he came just to bring a new religion, called Christianity, didn't make much sense to me. Most of the elements of Christianity can be found in other religions—the commandments of Judaism, the compassion of Buddhism, the forgiveness of Hinduism, the golden rule of Taoism.

The crucifixion and resurrection of Jesus is not original either. The Egyptian god Osiris was also said to have been murdered, and then resurrected to preside as a deity. Probably the least original idea of all found in Christianity was the idea of life after death in general. Judaism, Zoroastrianism, Hinduism and Buddhism all espouse concepts of an afterlife and all predate Jesus, some by thousands of years. Not particularly revolutionary.

I don't mean to offend anyone's religious sensibilities, or to conflict with existing beliefs, but to share my own experiencing. If we agree that Jesus was a revolutionary, where is the revolution? Because it looks to me like whatever Jesus was trying to impart to us, his interpreters have largely put him back into contexts that were familiar to them. This is the danger of being a true revolutionary who is martyred—without the opportunity to tell your own story, you're dependent on the wisdom of others.

"Your kingdom come, your will be done, on earth as it is in heaven."

— Matthew 6:10

As I binge-watched *The Chosen* and reflected on the ministry of Jesus, I felt like a veil was lifting. I saw so clearly that the Kingdom he was seeking to establish was in this life, not the next. This is the real revolution Jesus was trying to bring about. This means he wasn't trying to teach people how to get to heaven, he was trying to show people that we can have heaven here on earth, and that means immortality. More about the Kingdom and what it means in Chapter 7.

This is the truly revolutionary nature of Jesus—that he was seeking to connect people to physical immortality, not spiritual immortality. I'm not the first person to make this connection. Charles Brown first introduced me to this perspective in the 1970s. He spoke about this topic with incredible eloquence and power. Charles believed that Jesus was seeking to bring immortality to people and that was what got Jesus in trouble with the authorities, because they were not prepared to accept immortality as our true way of life, any more than most people are today.

There are numerous quotes attributed to Jesus about immortality. The Gospel of John is particularly strong in conveying this. Here are a few:

"For God so loved the world that He gave His only Son, that whoever believes in him shall not perish but have eternal life."

—John 3:16

* * * * *

"Whoever drinks the water I give them will never thirst. Indeed, the water I give them will become in them a spring of water welling up to eternal life."

—John 4:14

* * * * *

"Truly, truly, I say to you, whoever hears my word and believes him who sent me has eternal life. He does not come into judgment but has passed from death to life."

—John 5:24

* * * * *

"For this is the will of my Father, that everyone who looks on the Son and believes in him should have eternal life."

—John 6:40

* * * * *

I'm not trying to make just a scriptural argument here. There are a lot of things recorded in the Bible, both the Old Testament and the New Testament. Some of them attest to what I'm speaking, some of them contradict it. What I'm saying is that there is more to Jesus than what conventional religion teaches.

Of course, religion interprets these quotes to mean immortality after death. That is the status quo they operate from. But where is the revolution in that? Every ancient culture had its own ideas of an afterlife. Did Jesus come just to give another version of the same old same old? I don't think so.

To be clear, I'm not at war with religion or any existing ideology. But it's obvious to me that the ways we've thought about and organized life as we know it have not worked. It's not just Christianity, and religion as a whole, that has fallen short. It's Marxism, capitalism, socialism and every "ism" that's come so far.

We live with constant survival anxiety and always have. We may hold high beliefs about justice, compassion, and the value of human life, but under the pressure of survival people and the institutions that are supposed to represent them consistently lower themselves. We speak of peace on earth but none of us have ever seen it, nor is there any likelihood we will on our current trajectory. That's why this reconsideration now is of utmost importance.

Christians view Jesus as the Messiah, and I can see a certain truth to this. Immortality is the fulfillment of religion. By speaking of immortality, he was completing the purpose that is innate to religion, though lost in the clutter of rules and rituals.

I always admired Jesus, but because of his ultimate death, I realize now, I'd discounted his achievement. I thought that he had tried and failed to establish a new precedent of the value of human life. Not because of any lack of passion, purpose or wisdom on his part, but simply because the world he lived in wasn't ready. The Christians that were supposed to be espousing Jesus' teachings missed him just as the Pharisees had.

But I realized now that even though he'd been executed, Jesus hadn't failed. Because his words were fertile and in speaking out, he'd implanted this life in people. It's like there was this other life inside me, a life without struggle and survival anxiety, that somehow his words were bringing to life in me. If this sounds too religious, that's okay. You might say, I was having a religious experience about being alive. I was glued to this show, and the more I watched the ministry of Jesus dramatized, the more the feeling of calm and clarity grew in me.

But as I was watching, and more importantly, feeling, the inspiration that Jesus brought, I realized they had crucified him, but they couldn't crucify his energy, and this lifegiving, life-creating energy had gone into human beings. What he spoke went into bodies and has been carried down since then, and is something we all have inside us. I could feel this energy of life coursing through me.

As an immortalist, you might think I'm a dreamer. I would say I'm a visionary, but at the same time, I'm really extremely pragmatic; I'm most interested in what works. For example, I don't have an ideological attachment to naturopathic medicine vs. allopathic medicine. This dichotomy makes no sense to me. Because the purpose of life is to live, not to serve as proof of some conceptual argument. I just want the best solution for any given situation.

Many immortalists I've met over the years want their immortality to come a particular way. If they're into yoga, they sometimes want to believe yoga is the key. If they are into a way of eating, like paleo, they want to believe that paleo will get them to forever. To me, this kind of thinking isn't focused on living, it's focused on being right. I don't care about being right, I just want what works; I want to live.

One thing I realized as I was contemplating the life of Jesus is that the way we've been programmed to live by evolution doesn't serve us because it's not designed to. It's designed to perpetuate the species. In effect, evolution is a system of sacrifice, which feeds on us to achieve its own ends. No wonder, as it's written in the Book of Job, "Man that is born of a woman is of few days, and full of trouble."

We are born into a system of struggle and strain to get somewhere in life that we can never reach from within that program. Instead, we get the anxiety of failure and the supposed prizes of success that never really fulfill us. Evolution, and the social, political, and economic structures it has spawned, doesn't serve us. On the contrary, unless we have an awakening, we live our whole life in the service of evolution.

All the self-help work we do on ourselves cannot fundamentally change the reality of our situation. Yes, we may gain some temporary respite from our troubles, but in the end, our troubles always catch up with us, and somewhere deep in our psyche we know this, and we can never really let go to live. No wonder we die after seventy, eighty, or ninety years—living by the stress of survival is not sustainable.

We've all been taught to make the best of the life we've got, but how good can it really get? You might say, the more we try to survive, the less we live. But this survival is so deeply ingrained in us, that we end up playing out the same life we saw our parents live over and over, with just superficial modifications.

The good news is there's another life, another program, you might say, that is also inside us. This became clear to me as I was watching Jesus carry out his ministry. I don't think Jesus created this life. I think he tapped into it and came to embody it.

When Jesus wandered in the wilderness, it is said that he went out to be tempted by the devil. But there are different ways to interpret that. The word devil comes from the Greek diablos, which means, among other things, to scatter. Some scholars interpret this to mean the devil is one who creates division. I think Jesus went out to wrestle with the duality of being human that he felt in his body—the split between the divinity we display at our best, and the animal cruelty we show at our worst. What is unique and transcendent about Jesus, in my opinion, is that he settled this duality in his own person and abandoned himself entirely to his divinity.

One aspect of the series *The Chosen* that I really appreciate is how they successfully show him as a physical human being, rather than some abstract, spiritual being. As I watched the show, a kind of meditation on Jesus triggered in me, and it felt like a veil was lifting, about him and consequently about myself, and potentially every single human being.

What I saw was that Jesus' life wasn't about perfection, as much as wholeness, and this is a crucial distinction. If we say Jesus was perfect, then this sets him apart from all of us, because none of us are perfect, and we can never aspire to be like him. But the wholeness he received of himself in the wilderness is something that is available inside each and every one of us.

I saw that Jesus had broken out of the struggle of the survival life into a new life that had no struggle in it. That was his real resurrection. Not from the grave after crucifixion, but from the life that was hopelessly divided between joy and sorrow, gain and loss, divinity and humiliation. In receiving his wholeness, his body quickened from mortal to immortal. His words were potent and had imprinted this life in humanity, even though most of us don't know it. I knew because I felt this quickening happening in me.

I know, this is a lot to get out of a TV show on Netflix. But at that point, it wasn't about a TV show at all, it was about a communion with a life that had no death in it. Even though we're often accused of being egotistical for wanting to live forever, being an immortalist really requires us to get over ourselves and our egos, so that we can open up to everything that is lifegiving to us and turn away from everything that is toxic.

In a way, I had been training myself for this moment all my life, opening to the unknown, letting go of control, and seeking, ever since I was a ten-year-old boy going with my mother to hear all kinds of speakers, for the fulfillment of my hunger for life. Many of these people had some kind of enlightenment in them that enriched my life. I saw now that there was this bloodline that ran down through human existence of light and life that Jesus had made physical.

This lineage is the source of all inspiration and any progress in our humanity we can claim, and with it comes the energy of creation that is more powerful than any destructive force inside us.

As I watched, I was getting more energized every day because I was feeling freer and freer from what had held me down. I felt myself stop trying to cope with the troubles of the world and to defend myself against them. I realized I had often felt misunderstood and was hurt by it. This had triggered defense mechanisms in me, which could make me argumentative and sometimes it was hard for me to hear what I needed to hear.

That was all part of the struggle of mortality, a struggle no one can win. Like I had to be right in order to validate myself. But the more I took on this other life, the life Jesus had accepted in his own form and shared with others, the less I felt like I had anything to defend. I was anointed into a new life. It's the greatest longevity hack of all time.

That was about three years ago, and now this energy of life is stronger in me than ever. The joy keeps coming, the excitement keeps coming, and the revelations keep coming. I still see the problems in the world, but I don't get buried in them anymore—I don't sink into the troubled waters.

Here's an example. This may sound funny to some people, but I used to get very upset about how badly people drive on the road. I saw people make terrible risk/reward decisions every day that threatened their lives and the lives of anyone on the road, including mine. They switched lanes without looking, they made left turns across oncoming traffic, they swerved while reading their phones behind the wheel.

For me, this illustrates the sleep of death our society operates in. People see accidents all the time, but somehow, either they don't think it can happen to them until it does, or they feel they're going to die anyway, so why bother being too aware. I believe that in a matter of years we will look back at autonomous human driving the way we remember driving without seatbelts in the 70s, as reckless, naïve, and fundamentally foolish. But until then, driving is probably the most dangerous thing we do on a daily basis.

I used to rage about these drivers all the time, but I really couldn't do anything about them. Now, I just don't feel that reaction in my body anymore. I quit worrying about them. I drive with care and stay out of collectively stupid driving patterns, such as several cars crowding each other down the freeway. Instead, I just let them go by and feel my own relaxation to drive in the manner that suits me.

This was recently put to the test, when I was blindsided by a guy running a red light, as a I drove through an intersection. I was shocked, because it came out of nowhere. But I felt so calm in it all. I was just grateful I wasn't hurt, and that the other driver, a young kid, wasn't hurt. As I got out of my car and approached him, I could see he was filled with apprehension and fear that I was going to go off on him. Instead I just gave him a warm smile and asked him if he was OK. He immediately became more relaxed. We both agreed that we were happy we were OK and that was the most important thing.

CHAPTER 2

An Endless-life Crisis

"Come to me, all you who are weary and burdened, and I will give you rest."

— Matthew 11:28

About a month earlier, I woke up in the middle of the night, feeling troubled, I wasn't sure why. It was February and the wind was up, whistling in our window panes. Ilana was sound asleep beside me (she is a champion sleeper). Our dogs were sleeping with us that night and Isabella was snoring lightly. I tried to turn over and go back to sleep but something was bothering me. I felt this heaviness inside me, like I was carrying a heavy burden, and it wouldn't let me rest.

I couldn't fall back to sleep, so I decided, instead of trying to resist this feeling, I would go with it to see what was there. I'm a strong-minded person, which is a good thing if you are a longevity revolutionary trying to help bring about a massive shift in the human condition. But sometimes being strong minded can lead to over-riding what's really happening with you. Maybe that's why this hit me in the middle of the night when I was sound asleep and my mind couldn't engage to try to clear it out of the way.

I lay awake for about an hour and I probably would have stayed awake all night, but I realized as I lay there, that something had to change in my life. I didn't know what exactly, and I didn't know how. All I knew was that the way I was living wasn't working for me anymore. That's the first step to any transformative experience, the simple admission that we need it. And I knew I needed it. This gave me the peace to go back to sleep.

The next morning when I got up, and in the days that followed, the need for change in my life became clearer and clearer. It's as if I'd had my head down working so long and so hard on the super longevity and immortality movement, that I hadn't really paid attention to what was going on inside me.

People who know me know I'm a very positive person. I believe we should, and eventually all of us will, be able to live unlimited lifespans. You can't get much more optimistic than that. This energy propelled me to found People Unlimited, the most committed immortalist community in the world. This optimism also led me to create the seminal longevity event, RAADfest, and to run it for a decade thus far. I've spoken in a dozen countries on four continents, been on TV shows you've heard of and been quoted in the media. I've had a lot of success, and, more importantly, I have great people in my life.

But I found myself feeling like the strength that had brought me to this point wasn't going to be enough to take me where I wanted to go, which was into an unlimited lifespan. I'm a visionary but I'm also pragmatic and been quoted in the media. I've had a lot of success, and, more importantly, I have great people in my life.

I look at everything that impacts longevity. Many people view this challenge as a scientific one, and rightfully so. We need scientific breakthroughs to free us from the shackles of aging so we can live without the tyranny of death. But there is also tremendous emotional and psychological strength required to get where we want to go. We don't always consider that.

It was 2021 and the Covid-19 pandemic had hit hard. I had lost people that were dear to me. That in itself was not something new. All along the way, I've lost people I've loved, and it's always been extremely painful. Death never felt right to me. It never felt like something I could just accept. I dealt with it because I had to. But everything we experience is recorded in us, and maybe it had all built up to a breaking point in me, because I just wasn't metabolizing these losses like I used to.

It was more than just the pandemic. Bernadeane was my business partner, but also my inspiration, often my guide, but always my greatest support in life. She had been diagnosed with breast cancer about seven years earlier. We found ways to treat her that didn't devastate her health and she'd done well. The cancer was gone for a time, but then returned. I was confident we would beat it, but the presence of that cancer troubled me along with everything else. I loved Bernie and I hated for her to have to go through the struggle of cancer.

The truth is it's tough being a revolutionary, and while I still felt like I was answering the most noble calling there is, to end involuntary aging and death, it could feel like a thankless task. Those of us that have led the charge for longevity and immortality know that we're facing resistance that is built into the very fabric of our society. We've faced it all along. I started speaking on the subject in the 70s. Where we are now is much further along, but still the obstacles sometimes seem endless.

I've seen brilliant scientists with insights that could transform our lives struggle to get funded. I've seen our movement misrepresented in the media in ways that are simply unfair—like it's just a vanity project for people with too much money, when aging causes more suffering than any other factor in the human experience.

It's not that we hadn't made strides. In 2016, my team and I had created RAADfest, the largest super longevity event in the world. It was a huge success with over a thousand people attending and we've done them every year since. New collaborations have come out of it, and I know we've shared information that has saved people's lives, because they've told me. We hear the stories every year.

The science of longevity has advanced. We have much more available to us than we did a decade ago. Personally, I've done numerous treatments including exosomes, stem cells, Eboo, therapeutic plasma exchange and several others. But we have not had the signature breakthrough many had hoped would come by now. Some in our movement were giving up on this happening for our generation.

I understand their concern and disappointment. But the idea of leaving the horror of aging for the next generation offends me to my core. Not only do I want to live myself, but I feel a responsibility, which I know my colleagues share, to make the difference ourselves, so that the next generation can live in freedom as human beings are meant to. But it didn't seem to be happening fast enough and that weighed on me.

In my fifty years of being a longevity warrior, I've personally faced a lot of resistance from people who couldn't accept a new perspective on living—that we can have indefinite lifespans, and that this is worth pursuing. Sometimes it seems that people are so programmed to die that they are going to keep that appointment with death no matter what I say or do.

Working with biology in the lab is challenging, but so is working with people in real life. If you're not careful, as you try to educate them, you can take on too much responsibility for their choices. The potential for immortality should be the best news in the world. But some people just can't see it, and struggling to make them can cause them to react against you; they can turn resentful and even mean. I've confronted many people over the years. Sometimes I wanted to grab people by the shoulders and just shake them and say wake up!

I felt this way because I cared, but the problem is the person I was talking to didn't always feel the same urgency. They might think I was challenging them or putting them down. In fact, I was often triggering their unconscious will to stay exactly where they were. Change is personal. There is no blueprint for opening to a new paradigm and no profile for who will or who won't do it.

In all the years, I've never been able to identify what type of person is going to go with the new, and what type will stay behind. Some people blame religious training for the intransience of others, but I've met many atheists who are as dug in in their lives as anyone.

Some people say super longevity is only for the upper class, but I've met many wealthy people who took no interest whatsoever, and just as many people with little or no money who were extremely interested.

People can be exhilarating but people can also be contradictory to the point of hypocrisy. How many people have I heard say they want a better world, while they live totally contrary to what they say. They have their conversations about loving your fellow human, but when it gets intense, they go right back to the patterns that destroy themselves and others.

Working with people can be thrilling, when you see them transforming their lives, but it can also be exhausting. After decades of doing this, I could feel how much more energy and strength it was going to take to break out of this paradigm of mortality in our world. I still felt this calling and had no desire to quit, but I couldn't keep going the same old way. I asked myself: how could I really help change the patterns that are operating inside people to take them out of the struggle?

It was difficult to envision a world free from the horror and pain of the inevitability of death, to see it so clearly I could almost touch it sometimes, but also to see how far we are from it. It's not the scientific and technological challenges that bothered me, but the human resistance. I was frustrated with the slow pace at which our world moves. Here is all this new technology happening all the time, but where are the human advancements? How can people be so accepting of their own limitation when there so clearly is another way to go? The burden of it all was weighing me down. As an immortalist, I try to see the good in life at all times, but the simple truth is that there is too much suffering in our lives as they are currently constructed.

I'd always been a strong person, someone who could handle difficult situations and get through them. But maybe now it was all somehow bearing down on me, because I felt like the natural strength of just getting through life wasn't going to be enough for me. I felt like I needed to experience something I'd never felt before, something beyond just who I already knew myself to be. You could say I was looking for something supernatural that could help take me beyond all the troubles that were weighing me down.

At the same time, I also felt like I wanted a deeper connection with people. We'd built a community through People Unlimited that was exceptional. We had weekly events with regulars attending both in person and online. We shared a lot of love and passion for living, spoke freely about our intention to live without death and about the latest science and the clinical protocols. All that was good.

But something was missing for me. Despite all our shared purpose, somehow, we hadn't reached the depths of connection for which I had hoped. I knew that mortality is the source of separation between people, that the inevitability of loss creates a barrier that stops us from being as close as we could be. At the same time, I knew we needed that deep connection to carry us through to where we wanted to get to. Unlimited lifespans and unlimited human connection go hand in hand. It takes one to achieve the other; true togetherness is a vital component of the immortality equation, just as immortality is essential to greater togetherness.

So, this was a conundrum, because although many of us sincerely loved each other, we didn't really feel the freedom to connect at that deeper level. And frankly, I didn't always know how to get through to people. Sometimes I ended up raising their anxieties instead of relieving them.

The songs say, "love is the answer," but love has been around for a long time and it really hasn't solved anything. Don't get me wrong—I think love is beautiful. I love *love*, but under the pressures and struggles of mortality, love has never really had the full opportunity to flourish. We love and we lose and that is a source of great anguish and separation.

It's a chicken and egg scenario. Which comes first, the profound connection or the immortality? The absence of one was holding up the advent of the other and I had an innate sense that there had to be a way out of this puzzle, that we could create a connection that was so powerful you might say it was divine, a bond between people that could literally save lives.

I also wanted a deeper connection within myself. I wanted to know who I really was underneath all the experiences and beyond everything I knew. You can say I felt a kind of spiritual hunger to go somewhere I hadn't gone and be someone I hadn't yet been.

That might sound strange coming from someone who has been alive seventy-four years—we're supposed to be putting our affairs in order and preparing to die. But I don't live my life according to the number of years I've been here. If a person in their twenties talked about wanting to know their true selves, we might consider that an admirable thing. If a person in their forties or fifties was expressing such things, we might call it a midlife crisis. I guess you can say I was in an endless life crisis.

Limited lifespans leave us limited opportunities for transformation. But living an unlimited lifespan means it's always time to go deeper and to be open for more. Still, it wasn't really a crisis, and this is an important point. My life was good. My health was good. My intimate living was good. Everything was good but this travail was growing in my body.

The literal meaning of the term travail is hard work, but it also refers to a kind of inner working that can happen within us, a labor that brings forth new life. The key to such a travail is to let it happen. It can be uncomfortable because it brings up feelings we're not used to having. I think of it as a kind of tilling of the soil of our being, that turns over the old in us and brings up the new.

I allowed myself to travail. Rather than coming up with some quick, positive answer to cover up this feeling of need, I allowed myself to go deep and feel the hunger that was moving in me. That can be a bit scary, but it's also an opportunity to go somewhere new in yourself and that's what I wanted.

There is unlimited depth within every human being. But we rarely connect to those deeper layers. Why? Because we are too busy surviving to discover what is really inside us. Our evolutionary path has imprinted us with profound survival anxiety. At one time we had to survive predators like lions and wolves, as well as extreme weather conditions that threatened us. Most of us are removed from those kinds of immediate threats today, but we still live with the ingrained fear of losing our lives. Because we still live with death.

The irony of survival is that while it might keep you alive in the short run, it isn't sustainable. No one can live a really long time in anxiety, much less forever. Even if you could, why would you want to? Without joy and relaxation and pleasure and self-expression life doesn't have much meaning. I would go so far as to say that living in survival isn't really living. Because we feel forced to continuously make choices that don't really satisfy us, but are just about getting by.

The obvious example is financial survival, in which people work jobs they don't like that turn into careers they don't enjoy, just to pay the bills. But social survival is just as limiting if not more so. Early in life we learn what aspects of our personality people will accept and what they will reject. We learn to form a mask of acceptability, and we live behind that mask, often even with the people with whom we are supposed to be intimate. As a result, we never really know what is inside one another, because we have already decided that the deepest most authentic feelings we may have will not be accepted. This leaves everyone alone, suppressed, and disconnected.

No wonder so many people still say they don't want to live forever. The only way they know how to live is in this state of survival. Immortality takes us out of survival. When we are no longer worried about losing our life is when we can live it to the fullest, instead of constantly compromising on what really matters most to us.

Survival anxiety is a vicious cycle we have to break out of. But even though I had thought about this and spoken about it for years, I was really still in it. I was too concerned about what people thought of me and my work. I was too reactive to people and the problems of the world. I was too focused on what was going wrong rather than what was going right.

I had joyous times but not all the time. That might sound like asking for too much, but if you're only joyous part of your life, what is going on the rest of your life? I didn't want to be someone who lives for the weekend or for the party or for the high moments, because the rest of life is basically a low moment or even a neutral moment. But that was what was happening to me.

I felt like I knew a lot about other people, but had I really looked at myself and what was the real priority for me? Did I have something to say about how I move and react to this world, or was I just another victim of it? My whole life I'd moved to end this in myself and others, but because I was still reacting to a world living in survival anxiety, I was still living in survival myself.

I wasn't quitting on longevity or on anything I'd started, I just somehow knew that the way I'd done it this far wasn't going to carry me into the future I wanted to experience. In a way, this is entirely consistent with being an immortalist. If we live here for very long periods of time, we will no doubt always be taking on new ways of being. In mortality, adulthood is sort of a dead end. You grow up, you develop a certain personality, and you play out that same way of being until the end.

I always felt like there should be more for people, like we should not be limited to just one road as grownups, but that like children, we should have the freedom to develop ourselves to meet the next moment as it developed. I believed in this freedom, but I hadn't necessarily taken it on fully. And now, suddenly, I was so hungry for it and had to find my way there.

CHAPTER 3

Your Immortal Inheritance: A Second Birth

"A woman, when she is in travail, hath sorrow, because her hour is come: but as soon as she is delivered of the child, she remembereth no more the anguish."

—John 16:21

The Gospel of John tells the story of Nicodemus, who was a Pharisee, which was the Jewish sect at the time of Jesus known for their commitment to the Law of Moses. The Pharisees were respected teachers in religious practice, and Nicodemus was also a member of the Sanhedrin, the ruling Jewish Council, so he had high social status.

Nicodemus became fascinated by Jesus and the miracles he could produce. He came to Jesus at night, possibly so that his peers wouldn't know about it, to learn more about him. But Jesus told him: *"No one can see the kingdom of God unless they are born again."*—John 3:3

Nicodemus didn't understand how he could be born again, since he'd already been born out of his mother's womb. This seems a bit thickheaded, especially for a man who was supposed to be learned. But when we are faced with an unknown, we tend to reach for what is already familiar to us.

I'm inviting you not to do this. These days, most of us are probably familiar with the concept of being born again in the Christian context. This involves accepting Jesus as Lord and Savior, which is considered a spiritual experience, but also involves accepting a lot of church teachings about a lot of things. While many people undoubtedly have a sincere response to being born again Christians, it tends to lead them into the belief system of being Christian.

I don't think this is what Jesus was proposing to Nicodemus. After all, Jesus said quite clearly that he had come to fulfill the law, not to introduce a new set of laws. I feel that the rebirth Jesus was speaking about was a biological one, meaning a physical change out of one state of being and into another. Now we can't become something we aren't in the first place. But when we receive the right stimulus, we are capable of making massive changes, changes that are so comprehensive, so transformational, that we become like a new person. I know this because this degree of change describes my own experience.

Your Mortal Lineage

I spent decades introducing people to super longevity and immortality. I'm proud to say that along with peers including Aubrey de Grey, Bill Faloon, Dr. Bill Andrews and others, I have been at the vanguard of the modern super longevity movement for decades. Part of my passion has been to help people see beyond a life that is limited to merely surviving until you die. I've wanted to awaken people to live in a more abundant way with more joy and aliveness. Not only does this enhance the quality of life, but I believe it enhances the quantity of life, and that if we really want to break the death barrier, we also have to break through the suppression of death and the intimidation of death, in order to create a life that is worth living indefinitely.

These had been my intentions and I had put my heart and soul into my work. I haven't been perfect, but I was always sincere in what I was trying to accomplish. The problem is that we are all born into a world of survival, and we are all profoundly marked, you might say, scarred, by death. We live on death's terms. What I mean is that over the generations, we have been programmed to accept death, even as our heart and soul yearn for life. In some fundamental way, we are in a state of constant struggle, and we accept that struggle as normal, so much so, that the absence of struggle seems utterly foreign to most people most of the time.

Regular life is a kind of battlefield, in which on some level or other, we are just trying to get by. We may try to rise above this survival dynamic, and many people and many programs claim they can help you do it. But what I've seen over the years is no matter what I said or did, I couldn't inspire people enough or teach them enough to move them out of this battlefield.

It has nothing to do with being a good person or a bad person. At some point, the pressures of mortality build up on even the best people, and they default to their innate survival responses. This really became clear to me during the Covid 19 pandemic, which amplified everyone's survival anxiety. I saw people staying home, afraid to go out, even as the worst of it passed. At the same time, I saw people in the life extension community, great people, getting discouraged and losing hope for answers during their lifetime.

Of course, some coped better than others. But everyone was affected. The truth is survival anxiety brings out the worst in people. I've seen this in random drivers on the street, so determined to get ahead of my car, that they will risk life and limb. I've seen this in people who were very near and dear to me, tremendous people with real passion for life, and deep insight about it, who couldn't enjoy their enlightenment.

But what changed for me was seeing my own survival responses, in my frustrations and anxieties. Was I really living to the fullest? I realized that even though I was trying to inspire and enlighten people on immortality, I was still just sharing another version of survival.

I always felt that physical immortality should bring us out of our survival anxiety patterns. If you want to change human behavior, you have to change the human condition. But after years of working on this, it wasn't really happening. If anything, I was getting worn down by people, politics, and the ways of the world, and getting more and more entangled in those ways.

It can seem like an impossible trap to get out of. We are born into a world designed by evolution for the survival of the species not the thriving of the individual. You could say the life we are born into isn't designed for us to live to our full potential for energy, joy, health, and abundance. On the contrary, it's designed to bring us to the age of reproduction and parenthood, and then clear the scene.

How do we embrace a higher life of love and abundance when we are set up for sacrifice, not just by society's expectations for the roles we are supposed to play, but by biology itself. Even the act of reproduction isn't made to fulfill us as people, though many people try. Family can be beautiful, but it can bring as much worry and suffering as it does joy and aliveness. We love our families, but they hardly bring us relief from the struggles of life. For many, family is the single greatest source of struggle in their lives. For others, family offers a certain respite from the instability of human connection, usually with certain compromises baked in to the arrangement. But it doesn't break the chains of bondage.

I'm not saying there's anything wrong with this, only that, like every institution that has emerged out of our evolutionary journey, family is a coping mechanism, rather than a source of redemption. The same is true of education, intimate love, career, professional accomplishment, and religion, which offers a way out, but only *after* death.

Where did this pattern of sacrifice start? Some scientists and philosophers theorize that the first single cell organism opted for reproduction over its own immortality, and that has been the system of life ever since. Mortality became the price of life, and we've paid for our life with our death ever since. Wow, that sucks.

This is sometimes positioned in a more positive light, with the idea that reproduction allows for mutation and change, whereas immortality is viewed as more of a static state. This is connected to the age-old bias against immortality, which, conveniently enough, accommodates the system we've been stuck in forever anyway. The change that occurs through genetic mutation doesn't do us any good as people—it only operates across generations. And whatever benefits you think you may be bequeathing to the next generation, what you're really passing down is the same old sacrifice.

Plus, the fear of loss and death inherent to evolution tends to consume our more progressive impulses leaving us more stuck in our lives than ever. More about this in Chapter 6 Transcending Evolution: From Survival to Creation. Because right now I want to talk about the way out of this vicious cycle of birth and sacrifice.

Your Immortal Lineage: The Easy Way Out

If sacrifice is the basis of our life, how do we make the most of even the limited lifespan we've got? I don't believe we can. The good news is that there is another life we can live that is not derived from evolution and fueled by sacrifice and death. It is the life Jesus was speaking about, and which he manifested physically, and by going there, and speaking about it to others, he imprinted it in us.

Which brings me back to Jesus and Nicodemus. Nicodemus wants to know how Jesus does the miraculous. Jesus tells him to see the Kingdom, he needs to be born again. In this story, I saw that we are not going to be able to think our way out of our survival programming. We are not going to be able to learn our way out of it. This way of being is too ingrained in us and in the generations before us. The only way is to be born again, out of survival and into the life that Jesus himself experienced and spoke of. A life of abundance and prosperity without struggle, which is a life we can live forever because it doesn't wear us down or require our ultimate sacrifice.

I realized I was, myself, experiencing being born again. I could see that this wasn't a rebirth into a religious ideology or identification, this was something much more personal than that. I was being reborn out of the program of survival I'd received from my parents and my upbringing, and into a life that was also inside me, the life Jesus himself had chosen and articulated.

There are a lot of techniques out there for letting go of stress and trauma. My experience is they're good to an extent, but ultimately, they're just coping mechanisms that don't last. I wanted something sustainable, something I didn't have to meditate for all the time to get some measure of peace of mind. Nothing wrong with meditation, but one day you're in a good place, one day you're in a bad place. But this is different. This joy is sustainable. You're not going to have to rebuild it every day because it builds day by day.

Could it really be that easy? I have a lot of compassion for people trying to free themselves from what torments them. They try self-help approaches, religious conversions, psychotropic drugs, and many other things. It's called "working on yourself." But I've noticed that the more people work at being alive, the more they seem to need to work at it. If you're not awake to it, you can turn your whole life into working on improving your life. Well that doesn't leave much time for living, does it?

We've carried struggle into every area of living including how we let go of struggle—we make a struggle out of that too. But this reborn experience is different. This is an inheritance, something that is already in your body—all you have to do is receive it. In fact, the less you work at this the better. The phrase *no pain no gain* does not apply. This is yours. Your immortal lineage that is hardwired into you, right alongside the program of struggle and survival.

There is no struggle in this program, and no limitation. You're not a small part of something bigger than you, like in evolution. On the contrary, you're the whole of everything. No more wearing out your body to achieve your goals. No more choosing between prosperity and health, as many do. No more martyrdom to bringing about a better world. Because the best world you can bring about is the world of unlimited living that is your inheritance.

The immortal lineage has no struggle in it, has no judgement in it, has no trauma in it, and has no death in it. How can this be? Because it's not derived from our evolutionary system based on death, but from the unlimited energy that created the universe itself, which runs through all of us. I don't know everything about this inheritance, but I know it's there for us if we claim it. And the more we claim it, the more we discover it.

Is this immortal inheritance all we need to do to live forever? No, but it's a hell of a good start. Because for sure we won't live forever, or even extend our lifespans significantly, bearing the burdens of anxiety, the toxins of self-rejection, and revulsion towards others.

We need scientific breakthroughs and better lifestyle choices and everything in between. But this immortal lineage gives us the emotional and psychological platform that allows us to accept our unlimited potential and pursue it with full, joyful hearts, rather than plodding through our own resistance and fear.

Whether we realize it or not, we've been trained to live in waiting. Waiting for what? Some kind of satisfaction, some relief from the stress of surviving. We try to find this relief in different ways. Some have sought this through material success, but then when they achieve it, they may feel more secure, but they are never fully liberated.

Many look to rituals like weddings and birthdays to feel elevated above the mundane struggle. But those moments don't last. Often, they become a source of worry themselves. Think of how big a deal people try to make out of their birthdays. But even if you have the best birthday in the world, whatever that is, it's still only one day. What about the rest of the year? Because this experience of wholeness and peace is so elusive, many are willing to wait until after death to have it, when they get to heaven.

But through being born again, into the immortal lineage that is already in us, we can experience our redemption now. It's not about life after death, it's about life *before* death, meaning right now. We are no longer on the outside of living looking in. When the immortal spirit inside you is quickened, you can feel a new energy, an energy that is not designed for survival, but for creation. This is the energy that formed the universe, and it's flowing in you if you'll let it. Because it's already yours.

We're programmed to have to labor for anything that's of worth; to earn every crumb we gain in life. But I'm saying that the most valuable thing we could ever attain is already ours. People say the most valuable thing is life itself, and of course, there is a truth to that. Yes, our life is invaluable, but because of the survival program that has been inscribed in us, we never get to fully enjoy life, at least not very much. The most valuable thing you've got isn't your life as is, it's the immortal inheritance already inscribed in you, which allows you to live without struggle.

The Roger Bannister of Immortality

I'm not afraid to say that I praise Jesus for this. He went there. He went to that place in his body of total wholeness, total acceptance of the value of his flesh, and consequently, of every single person he knew and those he met along the way. You might say that Jesus was the Roger Bannister of immortality.

Roger Bannister was the English runner who, on May 6, 1954, in Oxford became the first person in recorded history to run a mile in under four minutes. Until Bannister, many considered it to be an impossibility. Some argued that running a mile in less than four minutes would cause the human body to literally explode. When Bannister broke the four-minute mile barrier, it was a huge psychological breakthrough as well as an athletic one. Indeed, after he ran a mile in under four minutes, several others did the same and now it is commonplace.

Jesus didn't live forever. Tragically, we know he was executed, because he lived in a time when there was no tolerance for his revolutionary views. But despite the fact of his death, I feel like he still succeeded by rising above the mundane life of survival in himself, and embracing the divinity of being human. Like Roger Bannister set a new precedent for physical performance, you can say that Jesus set a new precedent for all of us to experience who we are when we're not under the shadow of death.

It's important to understand that this immortal inheritance isn't just recorded in certain texts of the New Testament. It's imprinted in our bodies, waiting for us to bear witness to it, so we can live this life ourselves.

I feel that Jesus started a new way of life, a living without death. It is awful that he was killed for this by people who didn't understand him and viewed him as a threat to their power. But it doesn't change the fact that Jesus manifested this energy of life unpolluted by the touch of death, and that he communicated it to others.

With Roger Bannister, the achievement was an obvious one. They timed him running a mile and he came in at 3 minutes 59.4 seconds. That was a close one! But Jesus' achievement has been veiled from our sight. He never had the opportunity to tell his own story fully. There was no freedom of expression in his time. He had to speak in parables to protect against accusations of blasphemy, which would have silenced him even sooner.

Consequently, his message has been left up to the interpretation of others. His disciples loved him, but they understood him only partially or not at all. Even so, according to early Christian writings, they were martyred as well, and thus their story has been told by others too. As a result, we have versions of Jesus that are filtered through the experiences of people who never knew or understood him. This is how Christianity can glorify his execution, when really it is his life that deserves the glory.

The Legacy of Jesus

People inherit wealth from their relatives all the time. They don't have to work for that inheritance, it's theirs. Sometimes that inheritance was created before the person was even born by someone they may never have known. They don't have to labor for that inheritance; it is simply theirs. This is the case with your immortal inheritance.

As I started to accept my immortal lineage, it moved my spirit deeply, but it was, and continues to be, a fully physical experience. I shifted out of a life centered on survival and into the life of creativity. I know now that I can move fully from my inspiration. Not just in moments when everything seems to be going well, which gives me confidence or validates my inspiration, but all the time. There is an energy of life running in my body that I never have to crucify. I can live by this energy of creation rather than being driven by the fear of loss.

In contrast to the deep patterning of evolution, in this immortal inheritance there is no sacrifice. I don't have to sacrifice my life for money or love, and certainly not for immortality. I no longer feel like I have to prove anything to anyone. That's the world of survival, where no one's really good enough, and everyone is constantly on trial, struggling to prove they are, which is why life itself becomes a trial.

The fear has left me. I'm no longer afraid of just being who I really am. People want to make a lot of money and are dying to do it. They struggle to leave a legacy or maybe become a famous person, but there is much more than that for us. We've been so busy trying to be something, we don't even really know who we are.

The immortal lineage takes us off death row. We're not sinners awaiting our sentencing. We may have made mistakes in our lives, but that doesn't mean we are sinners. In the immortal lineage there is no abuse and there is no sin. Because we are not living under the scarcity of death, we are not driven to struggle with others for what is theirs. We can be strong but also gentle. The lion in us can lie down with the lamb.

I can put my body first, and all things will be added on to me. Instead of thinking about how to make more money, I think: how can I be more alive. How can I best expand the development of my body in order to bless my life and the life of others.

Most of us have had moments of profound insight that came right out of our bodies. You might call that a gut feeling, but it's really more than that. It's your immortal lineage talking to you. I believe we've felt it in certain instances, but too often we allow the pressures of daily life to drown out that sound of life. Now, in this rebirth, I know I don't have to muffle that immortal spirit anymore.

I don't worship my body, but I do worship the intelligence of my body that is connected to this immortal inheritance. I listen to it now and seek to express it at every opportunity. I feel like I've been born out of the struggle. I'm excited about the life of creativity, of living to expand the development of my body, and receiving all the blessings that come with that. This is not a new idea. Prophets have been speaking about this forever. What's new is living it.

Your first birth happens when your father's sperm fertilizes the egg inside your mother. It's that physical, and we're grateful for it, because that's how we come into being. But your rebirth is also physical. It's when the immortal potential that is innate in every single person, which is waiting in a dormant state within you, is awoken by this spirit of life, that brings that potential to life.

I feel like the immortal potential in me was made fertile by the expressions of Jesus. In his case, I believe that Jesus drew on the immortal lineage that is found in the Jewish tradition to become awake himself. Beginning with the Tree of Life in Genesis, which was associated with eternal life, there are references to immortality sprinkled throughout the Old Testament.

Enoch, a descendent of Adam, was thought by some to have been made immortal, as was Melchizedek, who was supposed to have had no beginning or ending of days. Elijah is another touchstone for immortality. And the prophet Isaiah seems to have been a particular source of inspiration for Jesus, who said: "He will swallow up death forever; the Lord GOD will wipe away tears from all faces."

These are all clear references to immortality found within the Jewish tradition, but they have been largely ignored or overlooked. You might say this immortal lineage has always been around, but it's been kept under wraps, limited to side conversations, if mentioned at all. The thread of life was always there, but it's been interwoven so deeply with the fabric of survival that it's been almost invisible.

The fact is Jesus is a product of his Jewish tradition. He studied and took inspiration from the same sources as the Pharisees who declared him a heretic. You might say that while the Pharisees were eating from the Tree of Knowledge, which was concerned with the letter of the Mosaic law and intellectual interpretation of that law, Jesus was eating from the Tree of Life. The Tree of Life is symbolic of a direct contact with the divine and eternal life force.

The fact is Jesus saw something totally different—a kingdom and a divinity that was, and is, our birthright. He didn't just see this as knowledge, but as a physical reality. He allowed this spirit to penetrate him and make him fertile so he could be reborn into it.

He didn't come to introduce another religion to the world or to update an old one. He came to bring a new life, right smack in the middle of the old one. Rome was oppressing Israel. The whole planet was full of strife, just like it always is. And yet he declared that the kingdom is here now, a rebirth, a fresh start into a life without the tyranny of death.

As you're reading this, I hope to help spark your own rebirth, in whatever way that comes. What's important is not to crucify the energy of immortality you feel in your body. Whether we realize it or not, we've been doing this for eons. Now it's time to allow that rebirth to totally take place in our bodies, just as Jesus did two thousand years ago.

How do we do that? By feeding this hunger for life rather than shutting it down. By acknowledging this immortal lineage inside us rather than denying it.

I don't have any formula for you. There are no ten steps to this. You don't really even have to believe in Jesus. I'm not trying to get you to believe in him, I'm just giving the credit where I feel it's due. Nor am I discounting other great human beings who have tapped into the immortal lineage along the way before or since. We should be eternally grateful to every single person who has gleaned even an inkling of this life and shared it with others in whatever form.

You might want to take a closer look at the words of Jesus in the context of immortality. You might want to get down on your knees and pray. You might want to go out in nature somewhere quiet and just let yourself feel the life that is inside you waiting to be lived. There's no ideology you have to learn or agree to. Because this energy is already in your body and it marks the end of sacrifice for you, and for every single person who allows themselves to go there.

But don't keep this to yourself. Over the years, I can't tell you how many people have heard me speak on immortality, who told me they have had similar thoughts, but have never spoken them out loud. It's time to talk about our immortal inheritance out loud. It's time to listen to the will of this life and let it be done.

CHAPTER 4

Put Your Body First: What It Really Means to Live a Longevity Lifestyle

"But seek first the kingdom of God and His righteousness, and all these things will be added to you."

—Matthew 6:33, ESV

There's a lot of confusion about what it means to live a longevity lifestyle. Many people understand that what we eat and how we treat ourselves physically, including exercise, has an impact on how well and how long we live.

First of all, let me say, that's a big improvement. I remember several decades back a doctor telling me that what I ate made no difference to my health whatsoever. He said I could eat M&M's all day long and it wouldn't affect my health one way or another. What does that tell you? That we've come a long way, and also, you can't always assume doctors are right just because they're doctors.

Yes, eating the right amount of healthy food and getting regular exercise is important. But doing those things doesn't really mean you're living a longevity lifestyle. Because the key to longevity is sustainability. You may eat well and exercise and still be working yourself to death. Or you may be sacrificing yourself to some other cause.

Living a true longevity lifestyle means you're not sacrificing yourself anymore. This can be hard to tap into because we are driven by survival anxiety and programmed by evolution to sacrifice ourselves to something else. We may want to take better care of ourselves. We may resolve to carve out time to give our bodies what we need to thrive. But how often do we really do it?

Most of us are trained to follow a lifestyle of depletion. How this depletion plays out is different for different people. Some people sacrifice themselves to their career. Some people sacrifice themselves to social success. Some people sacrifice themselves to their family or a lover or a cause they believe in.

This impulse to sacrifice is so deeply ingrained in us that, ironically enough, some people even sacrifice themselves to what they consider their longevity lifestyle. They want to live longer and better, but they apply the same old sacrificial sensibility by training too hard, or restricting their eating too intensely, for example. Some people are wearing themselves out with their longevity strategies.

So, What is a True Longevity Lifestyle?

It's simple. A longevity lifestyle is a living that energizes you. If your lifestyle drains you rather than energizes you, that's not a longevity lifestyle. I can tell you what mine looks like, but that doesn't mean yours has to look the same. This life is in all of us. How we manifest it can vary widely from person to person. I'm not suggesting that you should copy what I do in some literal way, and I'm not a doctor. Always consult a trusted healthcare resource when you're making significant decisions about your health and longevity.

But I do feel great and I hope this inspires you to find what makes you feel great.

When I wake up in the morning, my first thought isn't *what do I need to get done today.* Instead, what I think about is *how can I energize my body.* This is what our focus should be. Whether it's how you move your body, what food you take in, or what thoughts you give your time to. What do you want to do to bring forth the immortal spirit of your body?

I like to give thanks for being alive. In that spirit of generosity, I'm not thinking about what is wrong with my life or wrong in the world. I'm thinking about what I want to create and the people with whom I want to create.

That brings excitement to me. That's how I want to start my day. I'm not bringing myself down with the latest trouble in the news, or what the government is doing right or wrong. The spirit of immortality in me isn't subject to the news. It's not about what's happening in the world, it's about what's happening in the world inside us.

That doesn't mean I don't care about my community and my world and about the suffering of others. But if I put my aliveness on hold until we get this world sorted out it will never happen. Does this world really need more anger, frustration, and worry? I don't think so. If anything, what we need is more people feeling the spirit and passion of being alive.

Think of Jesus. He didn't come in a particularly good time in the history of his people. His land was occupied by the oppressive force of Rome. Struggle and mistrust were everywhere. Yet he allowed himself to turn water into wine, which is to embrace the lineage of life and immortality that can produce virtue and goodness in the face of trouble and even evil.

When I get up in the morning, I wake up to a whole new world that is happening in me and in people who feel this way. I stretch out my arms to the sun and give thanks. I drink a glass of water at room temperature because we tend to get dehydrated through the night. Sometimes I add a little pink salt for electrolytes. I take a few different supplements for my digestion and a few other morning remedies. Not because I'm afraid of what could happen to me, but because I feel the joy of caring for my body.

I don't run to read my emails first thing in the morning to see what new problem has popped up. I'd rather check in with my body.

I wear a Whoop biometric device that measures the quality of my sleep through data points like resting heart rate and heart rate variability. This helps me verify that I'm taking good care of myself. It especially helps make me conscious of my sleep, and having a good night time routine that lets me wind down before sleep.

After using the bathroom and brushing my teeth, I do some stretches to prepare for the day. I'm breathing and moving my joints. These are simple movements that open up my chest and stretch my back. I might spend about thirty minutes on this first thing. Then I go to the kitchen to make black coffee or bullet coffee or sometimes green tea.

I'm not driven out of anxiety; I'm flowing with purpose. I'll check and see if I have any important messages that I need to respond to, but I don't necessarily answer them all at that time.

Your longevity lifestyle should build up your immune system not run it down. I like to take a product in the morning that supports IGF-1 (Insulin-like Growth Factor-1), which plays a significant role in immune system function.

It's all part of making time for my body. I don't put work and getting things done ahead of taking care of myself, because without me, nothing is going to get done anyway. The longevity lifestyle isn't just another to-do list driven life. We may think we're going to let go when we finish that list, but there are always more things that need to be done. Does that mean you can never relax? Unfortunately for a lot of people, the answer is yes.

We've been deeply trained to be a bunch of worker bees. As a result, much of our identity is wrapped up in what we do, what we accomplish, the status we feel that creates for us. But what we do is just what we do. It isn't even really us.

What's going to happen when we have machines that do most, if not all, of the work for us? That time may not be that far away. Are we going to be able to accept the blessings of freedom that come with that? Or are we going to be too tied into our worker identity to let go?

I'm not waiting for the robots. I'm letting go now. By being relaxed and feeling the joy of what I'm doing, I'm going to get a lot more done in less time anyway.

I like to check in with my team in the morning. I want to make sure they have what they need from me. But we don't just talk work—we take time to have inspiring conversations. It doesn't take away from getting things done. It helps us all stay connected to why we are working in the first place. I want them to feel as inspired as I feel.

I'm inspired to be alive. Don't wait to feel inspired about your life until you've reached some level of success you think gives you that permission. If you're connecting to your immortal lineage, you're already successful. What's more successful than feeling the fullness of why you were really born?

Some people are so proud of how hard they work or how little they sleep. One person told me they stayed up three nights to get a project done. Ok, fine. But guess what? There's always another project.

I was impressed to hear what the great golfer Scottie Scheffler said about his career before the 2025 Open Championship in Northern Ireland. "This is not a fulfilling life," Scheffler said. "It's fulfilling from the sense of accomplishment, but it's not fulfilling from a sense of the deepest places of your heart."

Scheffler said, "It feels like you work your whole life to celebrate winning a tournament for like a few minutes. It only lasts a few minutes." That's probably the best golfer of his generation talking.

What's interesting is that sharing these questions publicly about the value of what he was doing didn't hurt his golf game. In the tournaments that followed, he kept playing at least as well if not better. By taking the freedom to question the system most golfers seem to accept without a second thought, he gave himself some space to feel and reflect. This didn't hurt his performance, and if anything, it improved it.

Working with clarity makes things happen; Working through a fog just drains you.

We don't have to be slaves to the system to be great at what we do and have a lot of success. On the contrary, the best way to perform at a high level is to free yourself from the slavery of survival, so that your spirit can rise to the moment.

You're a human being. You have the divine spirit of life in you. That's the most important thing. Not the title or the salary or the to-do list.

It's popular for people to say you should work hard so you can play hard. I really don't see it that way anymore. I don't differentiate that much between work and play. I enjoy the work that I do. I'm actually playing while I'm working. Because I'm not running myself down, I'm not always needing time off to recharge myself.

I'm instinctively taking care of my body all the time. The work is much more pleasurable because I'm not working with a stress and strain that if I don't get this done something bad is going to happen to me. Or that the world depends on it. I'm not carrying that burden anymore. Jesus said he would take the burden off your shoulders and that's exactly what I feel now.

When something goes wrong at work, I don't love it, but I'm not subject to that either. I'm still in the Kingdom.

I'm not struggling with my work and I'm not looking to escape from it either. When I take a vacation, I'm not afraid to call in to my team to see what will happen. I don't want to be out of the loop, and anyway I enjoy talking with them. I have a great team, and they do a great job. But I'm not worried something's gonna happen to ruin my day. I'm not living like that anymore. I'm living in the Kingdom. I can be on vacation, take a call from work, and go right back to my vacation.

I like to work and to get things done, but I don't treat myself like a machine. For me the key is taking breaks about every hour. I might spend a few minutes getting red light therapy or just doing some breathing to be aware of my body and not get lost in my head.

You should take breaks from work anyway. Why not use that time to do simple movements that enhance your longevity. There is research that shows that spreading your workout throughout the day is actually more beneficial than concentrating it into a set hour or two. So I like to do exercises when I take breaks.

I don't just do weight training; I also do mobility training. Keeping our mobility is a big part of extending our longevity. Things like jumping and squats are really important. Another good exercise is standing on one leg and closing your eyes. This helps improve your balance and stability. Spinning is also important for maintaining good balance.

We all need some kind of structure and schedule to live by. I understand that. I schedule my own time too. But the structure isn't the point. It's not a law of life; it's just a tool I use to help my life to flow.

In general, I would say we have too many rules, and the rules themselves will wear you out.

We have rules about what to say and what not to say. What to feel and what not to feel. How to dress. How to eat. How to think. Trying to follow all the rules we've created, straining to not mess up—it's a drain. We want to do everything just right so that we will be acceptable to our social circles or successful in business or even just so we can accept ourselves. That is a lot of effort and for what? Don't we see that the people we are determined to impress are in the same struggle?

These rules become superstition that we follow out of fear. It's all part of survival anxiety. If you follow a certain time schedule, you'll get your work done and you'll get paid and you'll survive. I don't live that way anymore.

The longevity lifestyle isn't based on rules; it's based on creation. Jesus said he came to fulfill the law. I believe him. The immortal lineage in your body is the fulfillment of the rules, because if there was anything good in all the rules human beings have created, it was to support life. Well, now it's time for life to lead, not the rules.

We don't have to be perfect to be totally alive and to thrive. That is another big burden off our shoulders. Not by might, not by power, but by my spirit sayeth the Lord. What does that mean? It means life fundamentally isn't about effort, it's about flow.

The daily living of longevity isn't about being constrained by rules. It's a wide-open space where we can breathe deeply and feel a freedom that we never experienced before for our own body, free of the consciousness of struggle and sin. You're no longer identifying with how old you are chronologically, but by the energy you feel in your body.

When it comes to eating, I like the axiom that we should eat for energy. I've been a carbo-holic at times, which would make me five to ten pounds overweight. I tended to overeat when I was stressing out, usually about people. I would find myself overeating and getting into a food coma. I wasn't energized at all.

But now I feel like I've satisfied a hunger of my soul. I'm not eating like I used to. I'm balancing out more and feeling more energy.

As far as what to eat, there's a lot of information out there and you can overdose on that too. I avoid processed foods and foods that have been treated with pesticides. And I limit sweets. I really like the principles of paleo or ancestral eating, which I learned about from Dr. Michael Rose, the evolutionary biologist. This comes down to the insight that we're much more evolved to eat what was available before the advent of agriculture, which only came into being in the last 15,000 years. So, especially over the age of 50, we're better off eating what human beings ate for most of their evolution, which excludes grains and dairy.

In terms of my health, I like to do blood work to know where I stand. I think it's important to have the data. I feel great, but I've had an enlarged prostate for many years. I have to keep track of that. But I don't test out of fear. I'm not in suspense as to how my next test will turn out. I've been reborn into my body. I have faith in my body.

It's not about being careless or ignoring symptoms. It's about taking the stressors off our bodies that weaken our faith and drain our energy. We can overcome a lot more than we even think if we take all these stressors off to be able to function the way we're supposed to. This is how we can make being alive sustainable forever. Not by worrying our way through the week, but by feeling the confidence that we can face what we need to face to live.

Fun is important. I'm not a big drinker, but I do enjoy a glass of wine with the people I love. For me, it's an enjoyment and I think enjoyment is good for us at many levels. Obviously, you can overdo it, but drinking too much just makes me tired. Nothing exciting about that.

In the Kingdom, Feeling is Freedom

I don't want to be in a zombie state. Some people chase the buzz and even glorify it because they associate feeling nothing with freedom. But in the Kingdom, it's the opposite. In the Kingdom, feeling is freedom. I'm not looking to numb out. For me, that's not the purpose of having a drink. It's about enjoyment not suppression.

I don't do recreational drugs or hallucinogens. I'm not saying they're wrong for anybody else, but for me, I don't want to sabotage the high I already have, which is the chemistry in my body that's natural now.

Let's not leave out sex. Sex is so important. Because sex is a special touch, which you don't get from talking. Just because you're here longer doesn't mean you have to stop sharing that sexual touch together. Some people think this is normal, but it's really not.

You don't age out of sex. Something happened. What has gotten in your way? Maybe you have some condition that stops you from enjoying sex, but that could be corrected. You don't have to stop. You can have great sex in your 80s, 90s and beyond.

It's not time that kills us; it's the burdens we carry through time. When you don't feel sensual anymore, when you don't feel energetic, maybe it's because of all the stress you're carrying from the present or the past.

Another key to the longevity lifestyle is the deep connection with other people. Longevity is not a competitive sport. It's the ultimate collaboration. The longer and better you live, the longer and better I can live. This is the best high there is.

Human connection is the bread of life. Before I had my reborn experience I had good conversation with people, but now I'm having communion with people. It's the deep that calls to the deep. We're communicating to our soul now not just our minds. It is nourishing and enlightening to the body, and this communication quickens the immortal spirit in us.

The longevity lifestyle is done with other people who feel the same way about living. It's not a lone identity trip. That's why I started People Unlimited, the immortalist community in Scottsdale, Arizona, with my beloved partner Bernadeane, in 1996. I knew we needed a community to truly live a longevity lifestyle.

We've had great times and we've had not-so-great times. I know I've been able to help a lot of people. I also know at times I struggled with people. Sometimes I wanted people to change more than they wanted to. Sometimes I saw something for them they didn't see for themselves. This created stress for all of us and sometimes animosity. Even when we really loved each other, sometimes we just couldn't get on the same page.

I was dedicated to my work, but I worried about people. I worried a lot. That took away from the enjoyment we could have had together. But since my experience of being reborn into the immortal lineage, I don't worry anymore. I don't care about people any less. In fact, I care more because I have more energy to feel them.

But I know it's not my job to fix anyone. No one really needs to be fixed anyway. I used to struggle with people to change destructive patterns in their life. And sometimes it got to the point that they resented me for it. Now I realize that changing patterns is great, but it doesn't change the underlying program of survival. Without a reborn experience, we're really not going to escape the system of sacrifice we were born into. So, why struggle over it?

We've been called a lot of things by people who didn't understand what we were doing. At one time, that really hurt me. Now I know that's just how the world works. It's not just me being targeted. Everyone is a target of the toxic critical mind. People need to tear people down because they feel torn down themselves. Because they are. That's the system we've lived in.

I don't want to tell people what to do. I want them to awaken to who they really are. We're ready to experience a different life, which is the Kingdom Jesus called us to live in.

We're ready to answer the call of this immortal lineage in our bodies, and to live that lineage every day.

CHAPTER 5

The Intelligence of the Most High: Tapping Into Your Divinity

"I and the Father are one."

—John 10:30

The God issue is a controversial subject in the sense that you can't prove there is a God, and you can't prove there isn't one. I'm not going to try to convince you one way or another. But I am going to give you my point of view, not because I want to disturb anyone's beliefs, but because it's part of lifting the veil on our immortal lineage.

As I've said, my purpose in writing this book is to share an experience and perspective that hasn't been brought out in the open before. Our immortal lineage has been kept in the shadows, and it's time to bring it out into the light. And with that comes a discussion of higher intelligence, which has typically been associated with gods not people.

Part of the power of the doctrines around gods is they tend to operate in a mystery, which can't be disproved. These mysteries form belief systems that many times dominate or overpower truth; much the way gods are supposed to dominate and overpower people.

From my own perspective, I've seen that we've always created a higher power outside of ourselves to serve our needs. The first need was probably security. We've wanted to feel like someone or something was looking out for us. But even with gods that are supposed to secure us, terrible things happen to people all the time because we live in an evolutionary system that sacrifices all of us in the end.

It's also true that religious institutions have used the idea of a higher power outside of us to control and manipulate their members. They do this by assuming the role of the voice of that higher power, and then telling people what to do, in the name of that higher power. Many people find comfort and a certain security in being told what to do in this manner.

But if the higher power is you, or at least in you, it's a lot harder to use it to control you. Typically that's not where the higher power is said to reside, because then you would be your own authority figure.

People have history, and so do gods, and if you look at the history of religion it's pretty clear that we create the gods we need at the time to survive. For example, in ancient Egypt they worshipped Ra the Sun god, because they were an agricultural society that needed the sun to raise crops. Norse cultures, which were warrior civilizations, worshipped Odin, god of wisdom, war, and death. As we grew more, in a sense, sophisticated, we created gods to match. Like the Judea-Christian god, who is more difficult to pinpoint than Ra or Odin.

Obviously, this perspective goes against certain conventional forms of religion. But the Bible itself states that the structure of what came to be Judaism, which formed the basis for Christianity and Islam, and shaped our entire conception of religion, was never supposed to be. The original intention was far different than what we ended up with.

For example, there was never supposed to be a priesthood separate from the people.

We were all supposed to be priests in our own right, rather than having some people singled out to be intermediaries between us and the divine. In Exodus, 19:5-6, God says: *"Now if you obey me fully and keep my covenant, then out of all nations you will be my treasured possession. Although the whole earth is mine, you will be for me a kingdom of priests and a holy nation."*

But the people were too scared to handle the direct communication of the Most High One. So, they said to Moses in Exodus 20:19, *"Speak to us yourself and we will listen. But do not have God speak to us or we will die."*

Similarly, according to the Book of Samuel, there was never supposed to be a king, because the people were supposed to be ruled by their divinity directly. Their divinity was supposed to be their king. But the people couldn't accept their own elevated status, that they in fact were royal. They needed someone, who was just another human being, to be elevated above them, and to rule them.

But when they said, *"Give us a king to lead us,"* this displeased Samuel, and he prayed to the Lord. And the Lord told him: *"Listen to all that the people are saying to you; it is not you they have rejected, but they have rejected me as their king."* Samuel 8:6–7.

And finally, there was never supposed to be a temple, because the divinity was everywhere among the people. *"I have not dwelt in a house from the day I brought the Israelites up out of Egypt to this day. I have been moving from place to place with a tent as my dwelling."* 2 Samuel 7:5–7.

Or as it's written in Corinthians 3:16(NIV). *"Don't you know that you yourselves are God's temple and that God's Spirit dwells in your midst?"*

What if the real inspiration for Moses to lead the People of Israel out of slavery was this higher intelligence of life within him?

Even if you argued that such a person never existed, he at least existed in the imagination of people who told the stories about him. What if that figure Moses was moved not by some external god, but by his own immortal lineage.

In Exodus 33:20, *God says: "You cannot see my face, for no one may see me and live."* Yet Moses was said to have spoken to God *"face to face"* in Exodus 33:11. But what if the face of the divine was his own? Imagine the passion it would have taken to face the divinity in himself in order to free his people from slavery.

You could also understand his anger when he came back down and the people were already worshipping a false idol, a Golden Calf. Because it can be hard to get people to let go of their old ways and to accept that divinity is their real inheritance.

All along there was this higher intelligence seeking to guide the People of Israel, who are a metaphor for all of us.

But the people were too scared or too petty or too self-denying to listen or understand. They were the chosen people, but they couldn't accept it and constantly chose to follow the norms of other nations.

Which brings us to Jesus. What did Jesus mean when he said he was the son of God, and that the "Father and I are one." Was he saying that he was some kind of perfected being that other people could never be? Was he claiming divinity that his fellow humans could not attain?

I feel like he was saying quite the opposite—that the divinity in him was in every single human being.

It's possible Jesus himself believed in a god up in the sky somewhere. He might have felt like God existed in the way that the Jewish tradition taught it, but that the divinity of God also dwelled in people. He may have bridged the gap between the human and the divine in that way. But it's also true that he lived in a time where there was no freedom of religion or freedom of dissent and if he did not believe in God in the manner that was expected at that time, he couldn't just come out and say it.

The truth is we don't necessarily know what Jesus believed. He spoke about bringing the Kingdom of heaven here on Earth, meaning taking what had been attributed to the heavenly sphere and grounding it here in our own lives. Rather than separating himself and divinity from the people, he was setting himself up as an example to empower us to receive our own divinity. He didn't want blind followers; he wanted people to wake up to who they really were and who we really are right now.

Whatever his beliefs might have been, it's clear that Jesus didn't believe in a god of judgement and vindictiveness and punishment.

But the people at that time were so programmed for a life of sacrifice, just as people are today, that they could never have received this interpretation.

Does God want retribution for your mistakes? Does God want to incriminate human beings so they feel less about themselves and about their fellow human beings?

To me, this doesn't sound like the will of some divine being at all. This sounds like the all too familiar self-condemnation of people. It's human beings who criticize each other and themselves. It's human beings who've never felt like they were good enough. It's human beings who have been trained to sacrifice themselves for the sake of evolution since the beginning of the species.

It doesn't surprise me at all that we came up with a god who is judgmental, and frankly, lacking in compassion. Because our own death programming has disassociated us from the sweetness of life and the sweetness of one another and of ourselves. We attribute these feelings of judgement and falling short to a god out there somewhere, but isn't this exactly how human beings feel about themselves most of the time?

If God, as we've conceived him, is so great, why does he need so much of our attention? Is God really so insecure that he needs us to pray to him constantly to acknowledge his greatness? Again, that doesn't sound like a god at all to me. That sounds like a bunch of people who are disconnected from their own self-worth and they need to be constantly built up because they don't really feel the value of themselves.

Maybe if we felt more of the joy of life and the beauty of health and the bliss of connecting with people we love, then we would envision a god who exuded those qualities.

I suspect that if Jesus believed in God in a literal way, then that would be the kind of God in which he believed. Because that was the feeling Jesus held for himself and for people.

Either way, Jesus was an example of the passion that we can all feel and move in when we open ourselves to what's really inside us. When we operate outside of the indoctrination of death, free of the cruelty that is inherent to mortality, and the denial of the body, we are divine. This experiencing is the redemption of the body. It doesn't come from some entity outside of ourselves. It's ours. It's our immortal inheritance.

If you ask me if there's a higher power, I would say yes, absolutely. There is a higher power. But it's not about a God who is sending us a messiah. It's not just one man coming who is going to change everything. The higher power I believe in is a collective power shared between people. It's our bodies together moving in the divinity that Jesus implanted in us. I'm an individual. We are all unique and irreplaceable. But together we form a higher power that I believe can create anything we need to live. The same energy that created the universe is flowing through us.

In the Bible, we read about serving the Lord and the Most High. That's been taken to mean that we're supposed to worship some being that is above and beyond us, a mystery unto itself. But Jesus brought this identity of a higher power back to the body. He said eat of my flesh and drink of my blood and you'll have everlasting life. Obviously, he wasn't talking about cannibalism. What he was saying was: take me on. Take on the intelligence that is flooding My body and let it flood your body. Let's have this communion of life together.

The intelligence of life that Jesus surrendered himself to is in all of us.

This is the Lord we need to serve. This is the Most High we need to listen and respond to.

It isn't a lone identity experience. I've had many epiphanies within myself about this immortal lineage, but my greatest joy and revelation comes when I'm sharing and connecting about it with other people. That's why Jesus said, "For where two or three are gathered in my name, there am I among them." Matthew 18:20. I believe that's because this life is a collective one, and the glory of it doesn't belong to any one person, but to all of us who partake of it together.

People don't typically share this depth of connection together. We live in a world where people live apart from one another. We can say technology is heightening this distance, because we text instead of talking, and talk from a distance instead of seeing one another in person. But technology is not the source of our separation, it's just another expression of it. We have learned not to get too close because of the pain of loss and death. We have also learned to protect ourselves from the attacks of others. People living in survival anxiety inevitably see other people as a threat they have to put down.

But despite all our protections, nothing is sweeter than the communion of our bodies together.

It takes a closeness to ignite this spirit of immortality in each of us, and to manifest it here and now, so we can have heaven on earth. Think about it. By creating heaven on earth, we won't have to argue anymore about whether or not heaven exists. We'll know it exists because we're living it. That's the only real way to know anything—to live it.

I would say the same is true of a higher power. The only way to know it's real is to live the higher power that we are.

Who are we listening to when we say we're listening to the Lord, the Most High one? I believe this is a call to listen to the intelligence of our body when it has been quickened to life.

When this spirit awakens in us it takes us from a mortal intelligence, which is the program of struggle and survival, to an immortal intelligence, which sees no limitation, carries no trauma, and promises only good news. This creates a higher movement for us, because we are no longer driven by fear, but we are inspired out of the innate passion for life and for creation that burns inside us.

We don't have to see others as lesser, because we no longer see ourselves that way. When we give this higher intelligence within us the credence it deserves, as the Lord or the Most High One, we empower ourselves to live the life that I believe Jesus meant for us to live. It's very powerful when we let go and allow ourselves to be led by this intelligence. At the same time, it's not really about power at all, because you no longer feel like you have to force your way into life or love or abundance. This is an anointing that opens the way. The veil is lifted and instead of struggling and sacrificing to get what you want in life, you begin to draw on this immortal inheritance.

This higher intelligence has always been with us, but we've never focused on it, nurtured it, or lived by it fully. Now is the time.

Think of how long life has existed on this planet. The planet is probably about 4.5 billion years old by current scientific estimates. Life first appeared on Earth about a billion years later, that's 3.5 billion years ago. That's a lot of time. Now think about how few years we settle for in our human existence. It's nothing, a blink of the eye, and we've come and gone. No wonder we feel no real stability or confidence in ourselves. No wonder our society doesn't value human life as it should. We've lived a life that is just passing through.

But this light of life has been around for thousands of years, maybe millions. I've speculated that it might even have been in that very first single cell organism, which chose reproduction over immortality billions of years ago. Maybe that organism was under too much pressure from its environment to opt for immortality at the moment. Maybe it had to go the way of reproduction to survive. But we're in a different time now.

Think of how long this spirit of life has been lying dormant waiting for the redemption of life and of the body.

And now, finally, it's happening. Not because someone we can identify as a messiah is coming to save everybody, or that some power is going to come down out of the sky, or in any of the other countless ways that human beings have imagined this would happen.

All those images of redemption have been defined by our own feelings of helplessness. The source of our redemption had to be something outside of ourselves because we've been taught to feel so little about our own bodies. But now we are recognizing that the very power of creation lies within us, encoded in this immortal inheritance. We no longer have to look to a god outside of ourselves or a god within us either. It's just us, when we are serving the Lord, which is our own bodies fully awakened to living.

CHAPTER 6

Stop Serving the System of Death

"He has sent me to proclaim freedom for the prisoners and recovery of sight for the blind, to set the oppressed free, to proclaim the year of the Lord's favor."

— Luke 4:18
(quoting Isaiah 61:1–2)

Some people are born into relative privilege and some to poverty. Some feel fortunate about their circumstances of life and some feel like they got a bad deal. But we have all been raised to serve the system of death. I realize that is a bold statement, and a perspective most haven't considered. We tend to think about freedom and oppression in mortal terms. This leads to endless political arguments between left wing positions and policies and right-wing positions and policies.

There is no end to these arguments because if we ever stopped arguing, pushing back against the other side, we would be forced to see how inadequate our own political positions are to resolve human suffering. Instead, we go back and forth, back and forth, arguing the relative rights and wrongs of our convictions with no real victory available to us. We spend all this energy on positions that even if we won them hands down, and the entire world yielded to our point of view, which will never happen, but even if it did, it would not bring about what we truly desire.

This is the epitome of serving the system. Think about it. Who wins these never-ending debates? The system wins, because while we are exhausting our creative energy fighting over what amounts to crumbs of truth, the status quo reigns supreme. Not only that—it is never even challenged. In all the fights over class and race and gender, individual responsibility versus collective impact, secular empiricism versus religious faith, the system of death that engenders all this conflict remains a given, an assumption that runs so deep it is never questioned.

What is the System of Death and How Do We Serve It?

You may be a fan of our current capitalist system, or you may critique it. You may consider yourself leaning more to the right politically or you may consider yourself more of a leftist. What I'm talking about runs much deeper than any of that. We've had many revolutions in history, which were supposed to bring us freedom. Some of them brought some measure of relief to some people; many only increased the oppression or simply gave it another form. Because none of them challenged the system of death with one exception—Jesus.

We all have our own personal politics, and issues we support and issues we're against. But the root cause of the system of death isn't any of these issues. And it really isn't anyone's fault. There is no bad guy in this story to blame or to push back against. We tend to like blaming others for our troubles and thus we get into endless arguments about whose fault a certain problem is and who benefits from perpetuating that problem. This feeds into age-old conflicts about right and wrong that are really just another distraction from addressing the system of death.

Now people have gotten better at demonizing each other because we have faster communications platforms on social media. Now we can really separate ourselves from others without giving it a second thought. It's not that we shouldn't call out people who are doing wrong. But blaming people for what's fundamentally wrong with our world is missing the point.

We need to quit blaming individuals and realize we're all born into this system that will never let us thrive to our full potential.

Most people can't see this system because it is so big, and so familiar they mistake it for reality itself. But we live in a special time when scientific advancement is enabling us to question the inevitability of death. And with this questioning, we can begin to glimpse the outline of the system of death.

We can sense this outline in the current healthcare system. Patients don't like it. Doctors don't like it. Who does it serve?

You can argue that the healthcare industry serves the shareholders in the companies that profit from it, but those shareholders are people too, healthcare consumers, who are relying on the same industry to help them stay alive. As a result, they lose too. We can talk about reforming the healthcare system, and many people do, but we will never make it what we really need it to be from within the system of death.

What's wrong with the healthcare system is just a glimpse into a larger system that simply cannot value human life as it should be valued. Because of this devaluation, no one benefits from the system of death. We are all hurt by it. But if no one benefits and everyone is harmed, why does this system persist? Who is keeping it going?

The system of death persists because we are deeply programmed to serve it. You might say we are slaves to it. This slavery takes many forms from the actual enslavement of people based on their race or tribe or cultural connection, to the slavery to ideologies and belief systems, to the slavery to roles in society and even the slavery to history itself.

There have been attempts throughout history to break free of this slavery. We've had great seers and prophets who tried to show the way out, addressing one element of slavery only to fall into another, constantly repeating the struggle for emancipation, only for the slavery to morph into another form. But it's always there.

Let My People Go

In the Bible, there is the great metaphor of the people of Israel being freed from slavery in Egypt. Moses hears a message from God, from his higher power, his Lord, to free his people. And he leads them out of Egypt, but they never really stop being slaves.

The moment they face the hardship of the desert, many want to go back right away. Later, they wander in the desert for forty years, supposedly for the generation that bears the consciousness of slavery to pass away so a new generation can emerge free of that slave's consciousness.

This is an argument many make against immortality. They say we need death in order to cleanse us of the old and bring in the new. But death never brings what is new. Rather it only brings more death. This is the model we've been trapped in forever.

In the biblical telling, as the people of Israel approach the Holy Land after all those years of wandering, they send out spies to check out the territory. The spies report back that powerful enemies are living there, which they will have to confront. Even then, after all the years in the desert, some still want to go back to Egypt. Why? Because they prefer the certainty of the known, even if it means slavery, over the uncertainty of the unknown.

In the biblical story the enemy is Pharaoh, but in reality, the root cause of our system of death we've been enslaved to is evolution itself. Evolution is a mechanism that is driven by death and therefore by sacrifice. Evolution has taught us that sacrifice is the only way forward, the only way to live. We see people sacrifice their health for money, their joy for acceptance, their creativity for security, and on and on. The best biomarker for how much you're serving the system is how much sacrifice you've got going on in your life.

The Program of Sacrifice

Sacrifice has been around a long time. Many ancient cultures sacrificed humans in the belief that it would appease their gods. When Jesus came, he said he was the end of sacrifice, but how clearly was that really understood? Was he just talking about the end of sacrificing animals at the Temple?

Most of us have been trained to sacrifice ourselves in some way every single day. We sacrifice our true identity, who we really are, so as not to disturb others. We sacrifice our real depth and communion of ourselves with each other because of public opinion. We want to get ahead with our money, and we sacrifice our soul for it. That's not necessarily everybody, but it's a lot of people. And anyway, the system of death we've lived under forces this sacrifice upon us even when we don't want it.

It's not a matter of right or wrong. It's a matter that this is the evolutionary response for the survival of the species that is hardwired into us. Instead of thriving as people, we are programmed to give up our lives for the survival of the species. Even people who selfishly pursue their own enrichment with no thought of others are part of this system, because they have sacrificed their feeling for others to get ahead, and without that feeling of connection and belonging they can never fully thrive.

One way or another, the system teaches us to settle for crumbs, both in terms of how long and how well we can live. A tiny percentage of people hold the majority of the wealth, and they're not actually happy. Some spend their whole lives to create their fortunes, then when they want to stop working to enjoy what they've created, they can't because they're too bored. We tend to celebrate this in our society for the work ethic it supposedly illustrates, but where is the real payoff for all the labor? We can't just enjoy what we've got because we're compelled to serve the system in order to value ourselves.

One way or another we get sucked into the life of sacrifice. A lot of people sincerely love Jesus, but they end up serving an institution rather than serving the life he ministered. Jesus proclaimed that he came to fulfill the law, but people let the laws of their churches take precedent over feeling and living his spirit.

People know that Jesus stood for more than these rules and rituals, but they don't want to be challenged. They don't want to be ostracized. They have a social connection they have to protect. But Jesus himself would never have let himself be tied to a structure that wasn't alive. He was constantly thinking of what is new, what is more.

There's no way out of it from within the system, but we keep trying. Trying to make it better only perpetuates the system because it gives us hope we can reform it, and turn the system of death into something that more clearly expresses our aspirations as humans. It never really happens, but we keep trying because what choice do we have?

Look at the hippy movement in the 60s and 70s. I remember, I was there. They thought their youthfulness was somehow going to take them out of the system. They thought they were going to start a whole new way of life, but it wasn't sustainable. They dropped out for a while, and rebelled against the status quo. But ultimately, they just became another version of the same status quo. Because they had some big ideas, but they never exited the system of death itself.

When you're stuck in a rut it's very hard to see anything else because you're used to going down that track. We've been indoctrinated by the system we keep trying to reform. We think if we elect a new president or bring in a new kind of government that will change everything. But it never does. Because it's not about really about the government, it's about the system of survival we have lived under for as long as anyone can remember.

A New Awakening

Within the system of death, you're always in anxiety. You may rise above the troubled waters at certain moments, but it's always temporary. You worry about where your next dollar is coming from. You worry about your health. You worry about what everybody thinks all the time. You're a slave of public opinion.

But now there is a new awakening that frees us from this system. There is an awakening to another lineage. We were born into this lineage of survival and sacrifice, of service to a system of death. But there's another lineage that has no sacrifice in it and that's what Jesus was speaking about and bringing to people. Jesus struck the note of freedom. By experiencing the divinity of his own body, he was able to hit the mark with others. He quotes from the prophet Isaiah, saying, "He has sent me to proclaim freedom for the prisoners."

Who are the prisoners? The poor suffering at the hands of the rich? The Jews suffering at the hands of the Romans? The women being oppressed by the men?

The prisoners are every single human being living the lineage of struggle and survival. Jesus proclaimed that the kingdom is here now, meaning we can live free now. We can end the slavery once and for all. We don't have to wait for a messiah to appear or for some magical external happening to occur. That's been our belief system, which has kept us on the hook, waiting. Jesus was saying the magic, the divinity, is ours. It's within us. We've looked everywhere else. When are we going to look within and see we no longer have to sacrifice ourselves and others.

Some say that Jesus whipped the money changers out of the outer court of the Temple because they were defiling it with commerce. In other words, because they were making money off of a sacred ritual. But it wasn't the money-making that offended him, it was the sacrifice. They were still selling animals for sacrifice right there at the Temple. He saw how pagan it was and he was frustrated that he wasn't being heard. I can imagine how he felt. I have felt that way at times myself. I think anybody that's really moving to create a better world for everyone and is blocked by the system has felt this way. The difference is that Jesus did make the difference. He set a new precedent and imprinted it in humanity.

So long as we are defined by mortality, so long as we are disposable and we experience others as disposable, then we are slaves to sacrifice, and we will never fulfill our divine potential. But Jesus said, *"Is it not written in your Law, 'I have said you are gods'?"* —John 10:34–36. As was often the case, he was referencing a traditional source, Psalm 82:6, in which God says, *"I said, you are gods, sons of the Most High."*

Jesus looked at the same teachings everyone else studied and saw something entirely different. How? By stepping out of the system of death and sacrifice to receive his own divinity and the divinity of others. Many of us are familiar with the idea, stated in Genesis 1:27, that we are made in the image of the divine, *"So God created mankind in his own image, in the image of God he created them; male and female he created them."*

Many people have read this to mean that we should treat others charitably or with some measure of value, which is nice, but that's hardly the real implication here. Do believers treat their god charitably? Do they admit that that entity has some value and should not be treated with contempt or abuse? No, they adore their god. They worship their god. This is the passion Jesus brought to people. We can say this is because of the greatness and the goodness of Jesus, which is certainly true. But that's not what he was actually trying to teach people.

What he was imprinting people with was *their* worthiness—that they were worthy of his adoration. That we all are. Not because of our status in society, or our knowledge or even our good deeds—but by virtue of being human beings. Many like to exalt Jesus and rightfully so, but it wasn't just about him at all, but about them, about us. All of us. Yes, he had a beautiful desire to uplift people. But it came from his ability to witness the absolute value of every person. It is this valuing that marks the end of sacrifice, and consequently freedom from the system of death.

Even when he was about he to be executed, he was still speaking of this wish for people to experience their divinity. *"That they all may be one, as You, Father, are in Me, and I in You; that they also may be one in Us, that the world may believe that You sent Me... I in them and You in Me, that they may be perfectly united."* —John 17:21–23

Let us now fulfill his desire. Jesus created a new lineage, a new genetics, for us to be reborn into. This isn't a new religious doctrine you have to believe in. This is a life already inside you that frees you from the system of death. It finds your value not in your sacrifice, but in your living to the very fullest. When we experience this absolute value of being human, we're finally free.

This reborn experience puts everybody an equal ground. There's no more discrimination between men and women.

Women no longer have to accept male domination, like they're under some law of punishment for being a female. That's all in the teachings of the of the old system. The system trains women to grow up to propagate the species. They are taught to fall in love. Love can be beautiful, but why *fall*? Why lose the sense of who you are and the value of your person?

People don't realize that love can be just a force driving reproduction, which has almost nothing to do with you as an individual. It's designated by evolution. It can start out feeling beautiful, but often it doesn't end up that way, because it's not designed to carry you through. It's designed to get you to have children and that's it.

But there is a love of the body, of oneself and others, that doesn't serve the system. You might choose to have children, but you're not driven to do so at the expense of your own life. You're coming together because you're interested in the propagation of new life in your own bodies. You're waking your souls up together. That love has energy that doesn't dwindle. It's sustainable. It's the energy that can carry us through eons.

The Freedom of Higher Purpose

No one has to do this. It's only if you are hungry to be free in your soul and you can't settle for anything less. Then you experience that you are the sum total of all things. You are the energy that created the universe. That's what Jesus was saying to all of us. Be the life that you are. Be that very energy of creation. That's what he was in his own body.

He wasn't wanting followers. He wasn't wanting people to worship him as something separate and apart from them, like he was the perfect leader, and they were the flawed followers.

He was wanting them to eat of his flesh and drink of his blood to become that very same life he was and be freed from the system of death once and for all.

That freedom is in all of us for us to tap into. But some people have resisted it for a very long time, or buried it so deep that they can't reach it. It's for every individual to make their own decision. I can't make that choice for you. I can't decide in advance who I think will have this awakening and who won't. I can't discriminate in that way. That's why I wrote this book—to give as many people as possible this opportunity.

When Jesus had this awakening, his brothers didn't like it. They thought he was nuts. For one thing, he was totally different from them and they couldn't handle that. Familiarity breeds contempt and they felt like they knew who he really was before he went out in the wilderness and surrendered to his true being. How could he be this person operating outside of the system?

It wasn't just his family who didn't understand. No one really understood, including his disciples. People who responded to him called him the Messiah. My own feeling is that he didn't want to be the Messiah, in the sense of being singled out as *the Savior*. Messiah literally means "anointed one." This comes from the tradition of anointing kings and prophets with oil to mark them as special. I think Jesus wanted everyone to experience being anointed, or chosen as special. This experience of being anointed takes us out of the system of death.

It's not about the type of job you have, whether you own your own business or work for a corporation. What's your purpose for working that job? Are you wearing yourself out for some goal outside yourself? Or does your purpose for your work come from your soul? Whether you're a carpenter or a heart surgeon, when you're connected to your immortal lineage, you've got a purpose greater than what the system is intending for you.

Everybody has some purpose in their life and that's a good thing. But they usually have limitations built into them. Our challenge is to get in touch with a higher purpose, a purpose that isn't defined by sacrifice and the system of death. I think that's what Jesus did. He got in touch with a higher purpose to bring this light to the world that no one had ever seen before. He had the purpose of bringing about the divinity of human beings. We had the idea of God's grace but he showed us how you and I together *are* this divine power. He had this willingness to discover who we really are and to receive the power that runs through us. Discovery is the purpose.

What do we have to lose now by serving this life that has been crying out from the beginning of time to have a voice? That's the purpose that goes beyond survival, to serve the Lord thy God with all thy heart and soul, so that all things are added unto you and that's what I'm experiencing right now. It doesn't mean don't make money. Or don't make kids. When you're serving this higher purpose, you're going beyond the will of the system, to tap into the will of your immortal inheritance.

We deserve more life as human beings. We need more time to discover who we really are and how to love one another without sacrifice. We need a new strength, which is a supernatural strength that comes from the immortal lineage. We have to admit that we don't have that. We don't have what we really should be having in the way of strength and vitality that is unending. There's a new spirit to feel and a new value of yourself to receive. It's not a sacrifice, it's a blessing.

I'm talking about total liberation. It's not by something you do or something you achieve. It's by the surrender to this lineage, by letting this spirit of life move between us. Jesus was looking for a witness of him, and in my opinion, he never really got it. But we can be that witness now. We can see that we don't have to serve this system of death anymore. That there's a new way to go. Amen.

CHAPTER 7

Training for Forever: Not By Might

"But he was speaking of the temple of his body."

—John 2:21

We need to move our bodies. We're made to move and we will have no longevity without it. But many of us live a sedentary lifestyle. Often, the longer we're here, the less we move. The less we move, the less energy we feel, the less we want to move. Everything decreases, except the guilt.

Don't worry, the purpose of this chapter is not to make you feel guilty about how much or how little you exercise. This is not about sin. Sin is the bureaucratic bookkeeping of death. It's how we measure ourselves and constantly find ourselves wanting. We've all done it and it's gotten us nowhere. Let's do this differently. Let's walk in the Kingdom together.

Death and survival anxiety have separated us from our bodies. Evolution has taught us that our body doesn't really matter, that we're just fodder for the next generation. And on and on. But Jesus came to reconnect us to our physicality, to remake the covenant between mind and body.

When he said eat of my flesh and drink of my blood, he was bringing divinity back to the body. Rather than out there in the air somewhere. You can't get much more physical than flesh and blood. And that's what longevity training is really all about—caring for your flesh and blood being on a daily basis.

There's a mountain near my house called Pinnacle Peak that I like to hike up. The trail is pretty smooth, and the views are beautiful. Once, I was coming down when a guy passed me on the run. He was probably in his thirties. A man walking next to me turned out to be an orthopedic surgeon, and he said, "by the time he gets to his 50s he's going to need a hip replacement."

Why would a person in their thirties be that reckless? Probably because consciously or unconsciously he thinks he has to go down the drain anyway. As the great baseball player Mickey Mantle put it, "If I'd known I was going to live this long, I'd have taken better care of myself." His father, grandfather, and several uncles all died young, mostly in their 30s or 40s. He drank heavily, and neglected his health, even though he was a professional athlete, and a great one at that.

Mantle was an extreme example, but mortality makes us all neglectful. If we knew we could live unlimited lifespans, we would cherish our fitness. We would never doubt the value of spending time and energy on exercise. Because we would know the return on that investment is unending. It would be crazy to let ourselves rot on the couch in front of the TV.

It would also be crazy to break ourselves down. But we're very programmed in our society that to push ourselves to the limits to get results. No pain, no gain. This starts with playing sports growing up, when you're taught to sacrifice your body for a result. You're a hero if you get injured for the team. Winning is what matters. Your body is just a means for getting there.

I played football in high school and then in college I suffered a serious back injury that could have affected my whole life. Fortunately, I was able to overcome that. But if you're not careful, you can pile up the injuries until you lose the ability to move entirely.

We think we have to lose it anyway, so why bother. But it's not true. We can get better with age. I just turned seventy-seven. I can't run like I did when I was twenty, but I feel great. I'm strong. I don't have pain in my body. I can move the way I want to.

Make It Sustainable

The most important thing about your longevity training is to make it sustainable. Remember, we're not just doing this for the moment. We're planning on being here for a long time. If you hate doing something, you're not going to stay with it. There are many ways to move your body. Find what you like to do. For example, I really don't enjoy running. I never have. But walking is great exercise, and I love to get out in my desert and walk. Walking regularly can be much better for you than hammering your body.

I also ride my mountain bike. I do resistance training. I play pickleball. Instead of trying to force yourself to do what you don't like, find what moves you and you could keep moving forever. But remember why you're doing it.

I love pickleball. It's a great longevity game. It burns calories, builds coordination, and sparks the quick firing muscles. I also enjoy the competition. It's fun to try to play my best and to beat the other team. But winning isn't the purpose of playing. My life and longevity are the purpose.

Playing pickleball the other day, I saw a woman lurch after a ball she shouldn't have gone for. She jumped for it and hit the fence and twisted her kneecap out of place. It was so bad the paramedics had to be called, and she was driven away in an ambulance. She's going to be out for weeks. It was sad to see, but everyone just took it for granted. As if getting injured is all part of playing the game.

Let's be conscious of our bodies at all times. Don't just jump into a sport and start playing. Do stretches and exercises to warm up your body. Play within your capacity. You don't have to get injured.

I don't go after balls I can't get to. And when I'm done, I'm done. I don't play past my limit. I'm not sacrificing my body to some external purpose. My body is the purpose. It's not that hard when you put your body first.

I hate to break the news to all the competition junkies out there, but when it comes to longevity, winning doesn't matter at all. Winning at pickleball or any other sport won't add years to your life, and losing won't subtract years. So, cool it on the competitive drive. A lot of that comes from insecurity anyway. You want to win to prove something about yourself. In pickleball? Really?

In the Kingdom, you're already whole and complete. You have nothing to prove. What a relief!

We're taught survival of the fittest, but in the arena of evolution and survival, no one is fit enough to survive. Don't worry about someone being better than you at a sport or stronger than you in the gym. It doesn't matter in the least. What matters is building your body to be more robust and resilient.

Please don't try to hold on to the performance levels of your youth. That's a great way to discourage yourself and even get injured. You don't have to be as strong or as fast as you were in your twenties. Think about what you really want to be able to do in life and let that be your motivator.

Maybe you want to be able to play with your kids or grandkids on the floor. Or to have good flexibility so you can enjoy gardening or traveling or other activities that turn you on. You should also want to build your balance and reflexes to live more safely and securely. These are real goals that you can work towards right now.

Last week I was going to take my dog, Marco, swimming in the pool. (Swimming is another great longevity sport, by the way.) There are four steps from the patio down to the pool. He was on the top step. I went to put the leash on him, but he pulled back, and I lost my balance falling backwards down the stairs. I thought, *I'm going to fall down these stairs and hit my head on the hard paving stone at the bottom.* I mean, I saw it happening.

I had the presence of mind to drop the leash and turn my body forward, so that if I fell, it would be on my hands and knees, not on my head. I stumbled down the stairs, but I never hit the ground. Instead, as I staggered down the steps, I was able to regain balance. My momentum carried me well beyond the last step, but I never fell over.

When I finally stopped, I stood there for a moment and gave thanks to my body for being able to navigate that trouble.

The fall was so imminent that it felt miraculous to avoid it. It helped that I didn't panic in the moment of falling. But I also give pickleball credit for sharpening my reflexes and stability while moving. That's the kind of result I'm looking for in my longevity training.

We don't have to get worse with age, but we do have to get smarter. The dumb things I did as a kid just don't work anymore. Stretching is a good example. I used to never stretch—I just jumped into whatever game was going on cold. Now I'm smart. I stretch both before activity and after.

Feeling Good is What Looks Good

Please don't work out just to look good in the mirror. We all want to look good in the mirror. But much of what we think is attractive is programmed into us by society. And because our society is driven by survival anxiety, any sign of aging is especially looked down on, particularly in women. It's not an expression of good taste or style, it's fear. How about just feeling good. What looks better than that?

Much of our attitudes towards physical beauty are clouded by evolution. For example, more muscle can make men look desirable to women, which makes men want more muscle. But those women may not even know that somewhere in their survival brain they see a man with muscle as being capable of producing a baby more likely to survive. They might not want children or even be able to get pregnant, but those triggers are still operating.

If you work with a personal trainer, it's important to find one that understands longevity training. Some trainers think it's their job to push you. They want to show their worth by impacting your performance. This can easily go too far. I'm really fortunate that my intimate partner, Ilana Lea, is a trainer who specializes in longevity training. She's very conscious first of all to not create an injury. Remember, the object is to build strength and flexibility without doing damage.

You don't have to lift very heavy weights to get results. I'm not into trying to break my records every week. Bodybuilding is not my sport, longevity is. The same goes with cardio and stretching. I'm not concerned about outdoing myself or anyone else.

The good news is that there are more and more ways to train for your longevity becoming available. One resource I use is OsteoStrong, a system for maintaining and even building bone density. Bone density is a big one for longevity. And they've figured out a way to do it safely through a series of machines, like leg presses, that allow you to max out your capacity without risking injury. And the whole circuit only takes fifteen minutes once a week.

Hang in there. More and more of these kinds of innovations are coming. That's why it's worthwhile to take care of your body now.

Another great tool is an electro muscle stimulation (EMS) suit. If this sounds like something out of the future, it is. The EMS covers your body like a wetsuit, and uses low frequency electric current to stimulate your muscles to contract and release while you're doing your reps.

There are several brands out there, I use one by Visionbody. Don't worry, it doesn't hurt. And you can set the level of intensity so it's right for you. This is a great way to train more efficiently. I can get a full body workout in just twenty-five minutes that would take four hours without the EMS suit.

It's also a wonderful way to build muscle while minimizing the risk of injury. For people who are already experiencing some frailty, the EMS suit allows you to train with little or no movement involving strain. You don't have to lift heavy weight or do an exhaustive number of reps to get results. I'm very thankful for this type of innovation.

The Numbers Serve Us; We Don't Serve the Numbers

I wear a biometric device called a Whoop, which gives me all kinds of data about my exercise, my sleep, the numbers of steps I take per day, and how much I've exerted myself.

It's important to have good data on your fitness levels. But I don't believe we should be emotionally enslaved to data. Numbers can go down but they can also go up. But they won't go up if we get too intimidated to do something about it. The numbers are for us—it's important we understand what our strengths are, and where we need to build more strength.

One important longevity biomarker is VO2 max. This refers to the maximum rate of oxygen your body can use during intense exercise. The higher your VO2 max, the better your cardiovascular health. For a while, my VO2 max wasn't as high as I wanted it to be. But since I started playing pickleball two or three times a week, my VO2 max has gone up about 20%. Now I'm in the top 10% for my age bracket and getting better all the time.

There's an assumption that the longer you're here the less mobile you are, the less flexible you are, and there's nothing you can do about it. But coming from the immortal lineage, I would encourage you to make the opposite assumption. Yes, it's true that babies' tissue is so soft they almost bounce. And we don't bounce anymore. But we do have the capacity in our bodies to exceed what we have been taught are the limitations of aging.

I know I've lost some physical capacity compared to where I was in my twenties and thirties. But that doesn't mean I'm on some steep downward spiral. Often times it's the comparison to the past that gets us down. I feel like we can plateau at a level that still provides us with the physical performance we need to fully enjoy living.

We have limited ourselves with our mentality about aging. The limitation is not in the body. It's in the program we run in our brains that holds us back. That program is always telling us that the longer we're here the worse we get. But our immortal inheritance is telling us something totally different—that we can be fresh in our lives, as fresh as a child. By manifesting this freshness in my body, I feel like I'm restoring the body to its rightful stature, and I'm having a blast doing it.

This doesn't happen by might, or by forcing some brutal workout regime on ourselves. It's about receiving the ebb and flow of your body. You're not struggling to be young or suffering old age. You're alive and sustainable, ready for the next innovation to come along to extend your life and enjoyment even more.

I take supplements to aid with workouts because they are good for me, not to try to manipulate my body to some higher level of performance. I take creatine every other day to build muscle. I also like to have a protein drink before working out and sometimes black coffee. I also drink electrolytes to replenish what I sweat out.

I don't like energy drinks like Red Bull. Too many stimulants can leave you burned out. It also causes anxiety. People on that stuff sometimes are the worst sports. They can't relax into the game. I like to win, but I don't like to be all wound up about it.

What does it really matter if you win or lose a game of pickleball? We're alive. We can move our bodies and enjoy our physical forms. We should feel flooded with gratefulness. Finally, we can come to the place of loving our bodies to the point we will do what it takes to care for ourselves.

CHAPTER 8

Transcending Evolution: From Survival to Creation

"Do not work for the food that perishes, but for the food that endures to eternal life . . ."

—John 6:27

We're not going to evolve out of evolution. That probably sounds pretty obvious, right? But it seems to be what we try to do as humans. We tend to plod along within this same system hoping we can improve ourselves or improve the system enough that it will somehow transform into something else entirely that can satisfy our appetites for living and loving and creating. But we never really transform—there's always something that draws us back to who we've always been. Because the system itself is not designed for transformation but for survival.

We can never discover how bright and joyful life can truly be, because darkness and suffering are built into it. We can never fully thrive within this system because sabotage is built into it. We can write all the beautiful songs about how love is the answer, but that love will never bring peace on this earth, because war is built into the system.

World War I was supposed to be the great war, the war to end all wars. But then came World War II. And immediately after that came the Cold War. We can point to individual factors that led to each war, but the truth of history is that there is always something that triggers war. Why? Because when the system is based on birth and death, death will always find a way, and it always does.

I'm not writing all this to depress you. On the contrary, I'm writing this to inspire you to open to something new, something unfamiliar. The familiar has always produced what we don't want. Why keep going that way? Why not open ourselves to what is not familiar but promises much more than what we've always known.

We are fortunate to live in a time in which science is starting to engage with our need for more life through the field of longevity. We are already seeing significant breakthroughs to extend our lives and we will undoubtedly see more. This will give rise to a whole new way of practicing medicine. Instead of standing by as the body grows more and more frail and eventually gives way to disease states that we treat with dead end therapies, we'll build strength as we go. A trip to the doctor will be to strengthen your vitality, not to mask symptoms with drugs and surgeries. Just like going to the gym to train the right way makes you stronger, going to the doctor will make you stronger too.

I am certain that at some point we will cure aging entirely. I know this sounds strange and even scary to some, but I feel this is exactly what Jesus saw for us—an abundant, unlimited life in which we finally value people to the fullest. There is no conflict between science and spirit.

As the Director of the not-for-profit Coalition for Radical Life Extension, I work closely with top scientists and clinicians in longevity. I hear from them first-hand the challenges they face. Of course, some of these challenges are biological. The human body is magnificent and complex. Now with the help of new technology, we can explore and measure deep into human biology to understand how to keep us alive and healthy for longer lifespans, and eventually unlimited lifespans.

But the biggest challenge scientists face isn't a scientific one, it's a human one. We still don't have the support and investment we need to develop longevity technologies at speed and scale. Investment is increasingly going into longevity and I'm grateful for that. But there is a lot of pressure on scientists to produce short term profits instead of funding them to cure root causes.

Too many people in power don't yet understand that longevity is the key to human health, and to advancing our society into a more just and joyful one where we more fully experience our divinity.

This is why our immortal lineage is vitally important. It's very difficult for people to accept that they deserve to live long, happy lives much less that such a thing is possible. And we're talking about unlimited life spans with vitality and strength. It's a beautiful new reality, which is so magnificent it can be hard for people to accept.

It's not anyone's fault. Experience has taught us well. The famous quote from the Book of Job says it clearly enough: *"Man that is born of a woman is of few days, and full of trouble."* —Job 14:1.

In one way or another, this has been the human experience thus far. But Jesus brought us a new human experience, an experience that is not corrupted by the stress and sacrifice of evolution.

When we embrace being reborn into our immortal lineage, when we tap into the life that Jesus manifested, we can experience a biological shift. We are no longer serving the system of death; we are no longer enslaved to that which will ultimately consume us. We are free to fully serve the life that Jesus spoke of, which is without the duality of life and death. This immortal lineage has no death in it and consequently has no duality in it.

Most of us don't even know what it feels like to even take a break from the stress of survival, much less to live free of it entirely. It's like the old cliché about trying to describe a television to someone who's never seen one—until they see it for themselves, they have no idea what you're talking about. Until you let yourself feel the freedom of the immortal lineage, you don't really know how good it can feel. But the difference is that this life is actually already in you. And it's waiting for you to open to it and to open to yourself in a whole new way.

The struggle of survival is normal for us—just another day at the office, in the relationship or with the family. We're so used to it we don't even realize how much energy we burn up just trying to get by. But let me tell you, when you let that go, you experience energy you never felt before.

When Jesus talked about how the Kingdom is here now, he was saying that we can have heaven here on earth right now. Some of his followers wanted him to overthrow the Roman occupation of Israel. Others wanted to fulfill different prophecies from the bible. But the Kingdom Jesus was talking about was the experience of our own wholeness.

We always put obstacles between us and the experience of our wholeness. We make our own fulfillment conditional on outside circumstances being just the way we think they should be. And guess what? They never are. And we're left wanting. We never enter the promised land.

But Jesus said the Kingdom is here now. Not because the politics were just right. Not because he was naive about how painful and dark life can be. But because his soul had awakened and he understood that the energy that had created the universe ran through him, and that in fact, he was the creator. As was every single other human being who shared in his awakening.

This is why we can't afford to wait for the world to be the way we think it should be to feel our immortal lineage. Only by surrendering to this sense of wholeness will we be able to create the world we want. If we wait, or try to fix the world first, we remain stuck in the web of survival anxiety and never experience that we can be the creators.

When you have this awakening, you know you are the creator. You're not reacting with anger or frustration or fear to people and situations that would have drained you before. And you're not subject to the public opinion of what everyone else thinks of you either. You can see what's wrong with the world, and even what's wrong in your own life, without bearing the heavy burden of it. You're free to walk on top of the troubled waters, rather than sinking into them.

When we stop living in reaction to the world of death that is when we start living. Because then all you're thinking about is how can you make this kingdom of life better. As a longevity activist, I feel inspired to work to make the world a better place for every single human being. What's different is that now I'm not waiting to experience my own divinity—I know it's already me.

We've always thought divinity was out there somewhere in some other place or dimension. We've never allowed ourselves to feel the magnificent dimensions of our own body. We've never gone there and that's what Jesus was speaking about when he said the Kingdom is here now.

How are we really going to have peace on earth? It won't come through negotiations. One treaty is made while another is broken. It won't come through education. Highly educated people have created as many conflicts as they've solved. It will come through a biological shift in which we accept our divinity and the divinity of our fellow human beings.

When we experience that this inheritance of wholeness is ours, we can stop reacting to people and that's when we can really listen. Someone might say something totally contrary to what you feel and it's okay. We can become more focused on what we want to build together, instead of trying to find something wrong with the other person. You can allow people to express themselves, to have a voice, which is real freedom of expression.

People want the freedom of expression to tear others down. We do need to speak for what we feel is right. But as long as we are just reacting to people, we don't have the full freedom of expression, because we never get to the point of expressing what is really in our soul. Our conversation is too crowded with reactions and counter-reactions. These reactions don't feed the soul, and they don't express the soul. They are just noise that blocks us from hearing one another and going to deeper places together that feed the soul.

Human beings are at the top of the evolutionary food chain. That means what threatens our survival is other humans. No wonder we have no peace on earth. We are programmed by eons of evolution to protect ourselves from other people, which puts us in perpetual conflict with one another.

It's only when we get out of this endless conflict that we enter into the mode of creativity. Instead of fighting, you want to build something creative with everybody you can. This makes us listen in a different way. We can dismiss the anger. We don't have to keep dwelling on what's wrong. Instead of tearing down other people, we can build each other and glorify who we are together.

When you're not in the struggle for survival, there's nothing left to do but create. I feel so blessed. I'm having these blessings come my way from everywhere.

It's a really physical experience. It's not some mental state we try to get ourselves in by following the ten steps to creativity. This is already there in your bodies. The work was already done by Jesus. He crossed over from survival to creation and set a new precedent we can all tap into. This gift doesn't belong to any one church or any one leader. It belongs to every human being. It's time to receive the blessings.

Don't struggle to leave a legacy for yourself—you are the legacy. Don't drive yourself to prove how prosperous you can be. Nothing wrong with making money, I'm all for it. But not to validate yourself when you're already valid by virtue of being a human being.

The chemistry of creation is a whole different dynamic. You're fueled by the power of creation that's within you, not to please some external source of approval. We've all seen these plants and trees that seem to grow through solid stone. How do they do it? Because the life force within them propels them to. That life force is what's both unstoppable and sustainable. All we have to do is unleash it.

I wrote earlier in this chapter about the challenges that longevity innovators face in attracting funding and political support. You could say that's the rock we need to go through and grow through. It's a long game to say the least.

Scientists who want to tackle true longevity are often pressured to deliver short-term profits. An example of this might be to develop some kind of wrinkle cream instead of developing a protocol that can truly lengthen telomeres. Telomeres are the caps at the end of the chromosomes that break down over time leading to degradation of our genomic information, believed to be a key cause of aging.

We need scientists that have faith in this direction and understand that their depth of purpose will attract the resources they need to pursue the real goal, rather than being distracted by short-term opportunities. This is no small thing. It's a big deal to stand your ground even when the marketplace tells you you're ahead of your time. It takes us getting out of survival and experiencing the divinity of our bodies.

At the Last Supper before His crucifixion, Jesus asked His disciples, *"When I sent you without purse, bag or sandals, did you lack anything?"*

"Nothing," they answered. —Luke 22:35(NIV)

Why did they lack for nothing? Because God provided for them? Not exactly. Because through doing the work of Jesus and moving in that divine spirit, they always created what they needed. That's the real power of creation that is within us.

Innovators face resistance. All of us who work in the longevity field know how much resistance we can come up against. It can make you feel like you have to compromise. But it's by staying on purpose and not letting that purpose be watered down that we have the power to draw everything we need to us. And sometimes that's very different from what we think we need.

We spend a lot of energy trying to fix ourselves and others. But I've realized I'm never going to fix anyone including myself and I don't need to.

I wasn't mean spirited. I've always sincerely wanted the best for people. But I would struggle to convince people to take better care of themselves, to reject the assumptions society put on them about age, to embrace their value as human beings. But I could never really make anyone do anything.

Now I know I really have no control over any of it and that's not a problem—that's a great thing. I have the power and authority to express myself and hopefully to stir people to explore this new reality. But it's up to every single person what they want to do with this feast. Your awakening is really up to you. If you want to break free from the system that has dominated your joy and aliveness, you can. Because there's a life inside you that isn't programmed by survival.

The rat race is real and so is the exit from the rat race. I've always taken time for myself to meditate and reflect and do things that build my body. But now it's just organic for me to put my body, me, my flesh first. When I find myself starting to struggle with something a little bit, I have a response in my body that says, hey that's not the way to go.

Not long ago, I needed to check some things in a safe deposit box at the bank. The bank person took me to the box but it was empty. There were supposed to be very important items in that box, which were worth some money. But the box was empty and the bank attendant acted like she knew nothing about it. She stood there looking at me as if to say: if the box is empty, it must be because there's nothing in it.

I felt worry rise in me. I knew there must be some mistake, but the banker wasn't giving me any credibility in the matter. I stood to lose some valuable things if this wasn't resolved. And we all know how institutions that make mistakes don't like to admit it, especially when it could cost them money. I told her that there had to be some error and asked her to go double check her paperwork that this was the correct box number.

In the time she was gone, which was a few minutes, I started to get very nervous and then I knew I wasn't going to go the way of fear and loss. I thought, *I'm not a desperate person. I'm not in survival anymore* and this very organic feeling came over me and I just relaxed. I released the whole thing. Whether my items were found or lost wasn't going to dictate who I am or my prosperity. I'm in the Kingdom.

Then the banker came back and I think she was actually kind of surprised. She said she talked to her manager who told her to check a particular file, where she found the correct box number, which of course had the stuff in it I had expected to find. Hallelujah.

I knew it had to be there and I was right. But I also knew that even if they didn't sort out their error, if I never got the right safe deposit box and the contents of it were lost, I wasn't going to lose. I wasn't going to go without.

What a great feeling to know that my well-being isn't dependent on any of it. What a freedom.

We have no idea how much our immune systems are affected by stress. And to be able to just release it, to live free of that scenario entirely is such a blessing.

I know to some people this sounds too good to be true. But if we aren't going for what is really pleasing to the soul and what can allow us to live longer and better, what is the point?

I also know that there are people out there who are tired of the old ways. You are tired of learning more coping mechanisms for a life that doesn't bless you and never will. You don't want to just put a band aid on a bad situation. You don't want just another variation on some old self-help theme. You're ready for the Kingdom.

Yes, as has often been pointed out by thoughtful people, we die alone. But to truly live, rather than just surviving, to live in the Kingdom, we need other people. In fact, I would say, for the first time, we really need other people. Because the Kingdom is experienced in a state of communion. Not with distant gods or invisible angels. But with people who share your passion for living.

We do have to get over our egos. What I've experienced, which is by far the most meaningful and transformative thing that has ever happened to me, didn't come from me. It came from another human being, Jesus. I'm not trying to upset anyone, but Jesus was a human being and it's his humanity that awakened me.

If he had people then who understood him, who received who he was and what he was trying to bring, the authorities could have never taken his life. If they treasured him instead of finding a way to get rid of him it would have been a whole different dynamics, because he was giving the bread of life out of his body. If they had partaken of that bread of life there could have been a whole new shift of energy within the whole structure of humanity. We would know our real value as human beings rather than settling for the crumbs that survival affords us.

I got this from Jesus and now I'm transferring it to you. I'm not the first one to connect Jesus to immortality. My former partner, Charles Brown, was extremely eloquent in making this connection. He changed my life. Others over time have made similar interpretations.

I can also say that Jesus wasn't the first prophet to connect to the immortal lineage. This lineage runs through the whole Bible in places. Many of Jesus' greatest pronouncements can be traced to sources from the Old Testament. But it's not limited to that.

The immortal line also runs through people not part of the Judea-Christian tradition. I would say every moment of real enlightenment in human history is because people were touched by this innate spirit of life, which let them look past the limitations of survival and into forever, even if just for a short time.

The difference is that Jesus went all the way with it. He made the word of immortality flesh in his body, and consequently we all have that in us. But we have to make the physical connection to someone who is fertile with this life. That's how it happens.

For the first time, people aren't just incidental to one another. In the Kingdom, we are vital to each other because together we share the bread of life. We're liberating each other from the death program. We're connecting with the Tree of Life, which grows in all of us, and we're passing these signals of life back and forth and our DNA is picking up on these signals and we're creating new life together.

CHAPTER 9

Faith in Action: What I Do For My Longevity on a Regular Basis

"Take up your mat and walk."

—John 5:8

In today's world, neglecting our bodies as we age is the norm. It takes faith to take action for your longevity. As you'll see in this chapter, I do a lot for my longevity. That's how much I believe in myself. Not as an egotistical lone identity, but as someone who has awakened to the immortal lineage that is within all of us. How much I do is a measure of how much I believe.

There's a story about a guy who goes out on his boat and gets caught out at sea in a storm. As the storm grows in intensity, he prays to his god to save him, he prays with all his might. Meanwhile a helicopter spots him in the storm and hovers above him to lower a rope, but he waves them away, saying "I believe my god will save me." A Coast Guard vessel approaches, offering him aid. He says, "No thank you, I believe in my god." A cruise ship passes by and wants to take him on board. Yet again, he says, "No, I'm waiting upon the Lord for help."

Finally, he drowns, and when he meets his maker, he says: "Why didn't you save me? I was waiting and waiting, and you never came."

His divine power says, "What do you mean, I sent you a helicopter, I sent you the Coast Guard, I sent the cruise ship, and you said no to all of them."

Let's not have a fixed image of where the blessing of our immortal lineage needs to come from. Longevity science and spirituality both emanate from the same source—the life force that animates us and moves us to create.

In this chapter, I'm going to share with you the protocols I do for my longevity. I'm not a doctor. I'm not trying to tell you what you should do. The purpose of this chapter is to give you ideas and inspiration for your own longevity.

Please don't be overwhelmed by how much is listed here. You don't have to do it all. You don't have to do anything. Just pick and choose what feels right to you.

Of course it's good to consult with a physician. The problem is many doctors are not aware of longevity, much less what you can do to support it. They look at you in the context of the average health and life expectancy of people your age in America. This is not the standard we want to set for ourselves. You can still consult with your doctor; just be aware you might be informing *them*. Unfortunately, most doctors are not trained in longevity medicine. As you're reading this, you may be more informed than they are.

What you won't find here is a silver bullet for longevity. Sadly, some companies still hype their products that way. The reality is no one product or protocol is available today to ensure your longevity. That's probably not even the right way to think about longevity.

Longevity is you building your resilience from whatever condition you find yourself in right now. You're a beautiful multifaceted person. You need a variety of ways to boost your life. We can't just take supplements. We have to cleanse ourselves too. The good news is there are many ways to do this and more answers on the way.

What I'm sharing here is not a fixed regimen. I'm constantly adding new things and taking others out. The science of longevity is moving as fast as the spirit of longevity. We need to adapt as new innovations become available.

The most important thing is that you start doing *something*. This will increase your well-being and vitality and give you more energy to do more things. But don't try to take on too much too soon. You don't need to win a marathon, when a good walk is enough to build your stamina.

Sustainability is key. Longevity isn't just another New Year's resolution. It's forever, and let's start thinking that way. Remember, we're here for the long run.

You don't necessarily have to spend a lot of money to get real results either. As you'll see, a lot of the protocols I follow are free, many are very affordable, and a few are more expensive. Don't get hung up on stuff you can't afford. Invest the time and money you can now and build yourself from there.

It reminds me of the famous miracle of the loaves and the fishes where Jesus created abundance for thousands out of just five loaves of bread and two fish. Don't worry about what you don't have or can't do. Don't drive yourself out of anxiety. Enjoy the fact that you are embracing your longevity. And let the momentum of your life expand exponentially.

Three Levels of Longevity Practices

I'm organizing these protocols into three levels that together form my longevity pyramid. I'll call the first level Cleanse & Nourish. This is the foundation for your longevity long term. The second level is Holistic Regenerative Practices. And the Third level is Advanced Longevity Therapies.

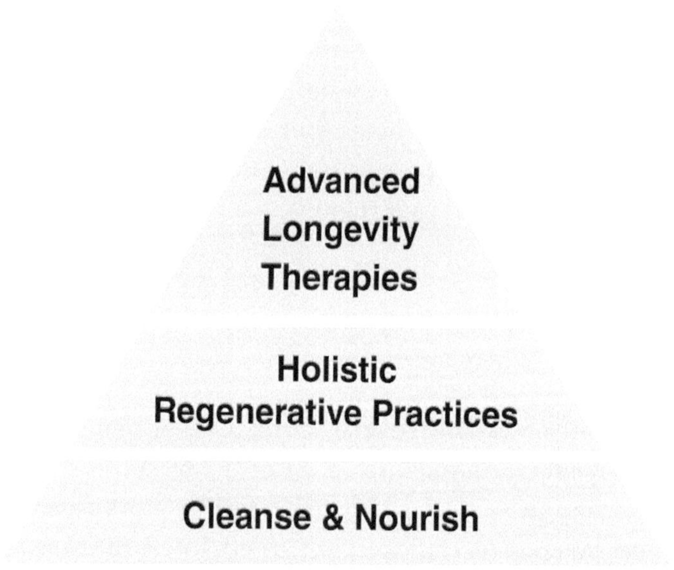

1. CLEANSE & NOURISH

- **Sunlight Salute**

  Right when I get out of bed, I walk outside to let the sun hit me for 3-5 minutes. This helps sets the circadian clocks in your body. It's a nice way to wake up and I never have to use an alarm.

- **Glass of Water with Salt**

  First thing, I drink a glass of water with pinch of Celtic or pink salt. It's a natural source of electrolytes, which helps control blood pressure, and keep the acid-base balance steady.

- **Drink Water**

  I drink water throughout the day. I aim to drink half my body weight in ounces. If you weigh 200 pounds, you should drink 100 ounces, which is 8 to 10, 8-ounce glasses of water.

- **Nitric Oxide**

  When I wake up, I take a nitric oxide lozenge, which has numerous benefits, including relaxing blood vessels and opening the vascular system.

- **Nattokinase**

  Strokes and heart attacks are sudden killers. To help bombproof myself, I take a natural blood thinner every day called Nattokinase. If you're already on a prescribed blood thinner, do not take both. But you might consult with your doctor to see if they will change you over to Nattokinase. I take 100 mg at night and one vitamin E in the morning.

- **Rooster Deep Breathing**

  It's good to boost your oxygen levels before starting your day and when going to bed. Ball your hands into fists and put them behind your back against your kidneys. Bring your elbows back to inhale. Then bring your elbows forward to exhale. I do the Rooster for 3-5 minutes.

Rooster Deep Breathing Exercise

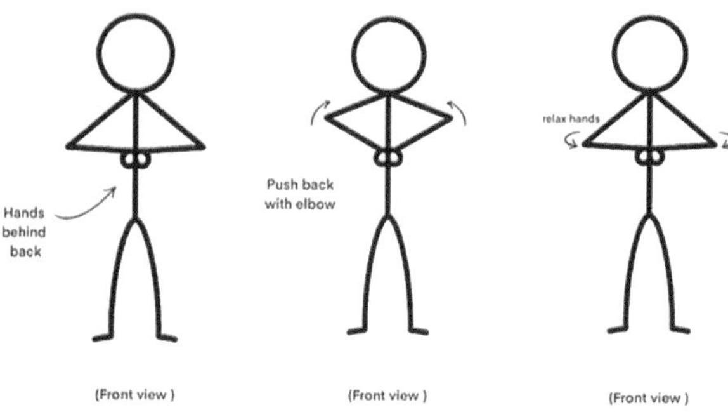

- **Bent Over Stomach Rolls**

  Wake up your digestive system in the morning by doing this exercise for about 1 minute. Bend over with hands on knees, roll stomach clockwise.

Bent Over Stomach Rolls Exercise

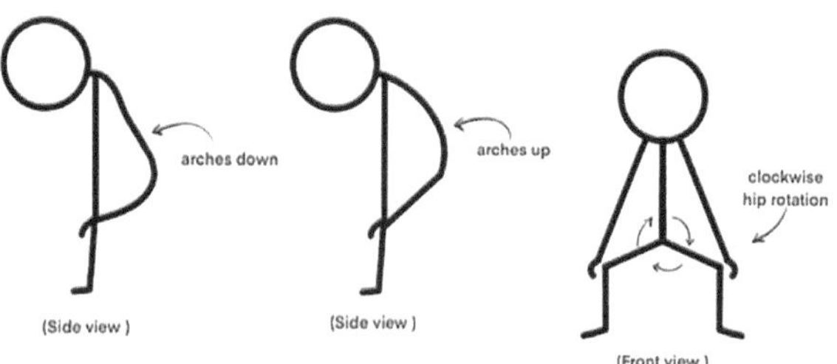

- **Morning Coffee**

  I use organic fresh ground, low acid coffee, and add 1 Tbsp. turkey tail mushroom powder, which builds the immune system.

  1 Tbsp. cocoa powder, a powerful anti-oxidant

  1 Tbsp. MCT oil, a blood cleanser

  And a scoop of collagen protein

- **Rebounder Bounce and Run**

  Rebounder is like a mini trampoline for grown-ups. I spend about 10 minutes alternating between bouncing and running in minute intervals. It gets the lymphatic system moving and strengthens muscle fibers.

- **Body Windmill Spins**

  Spread your arms out wide. Then rotate like a propeller. Start out slow and build up to 20 spins in either direction. This is fantastic for your balance.

Spinning Exercise

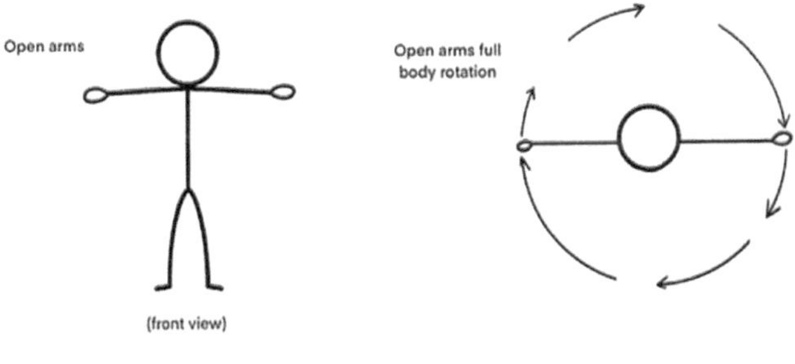

- **Neck Turns with Eyes Fixed**

  Focus your eyes on a point in front of you and keep looking at that point while you rotate your head left and right and up and down. 10-20 times in each direction. This is great for the small muscles in your neck, and for the muscles in your eyes.

- **Arms Cross Back Exercise**

  Spread arms with thumbs up. Move arms together and apart while alternating your hands going above and below each other. Repeat 8-10 times.

Arms Cross Back Exercise

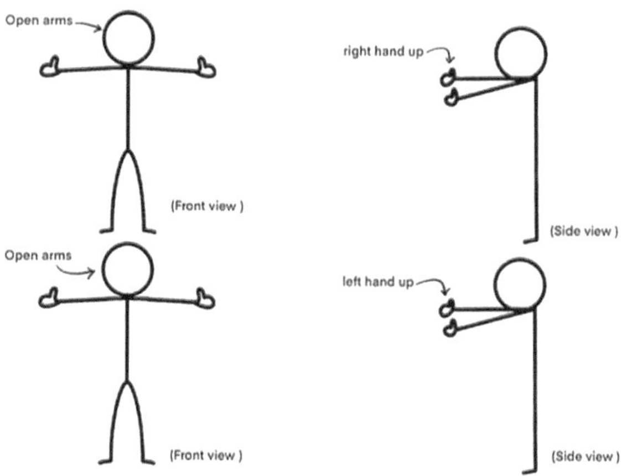

- **3-point Back Exercise**

  To help you avoid back trouble. Raise your arms in the air, bend forward at the waist and bring your hands toward the ground. Then bring your hands to your legs. Then bring your hands past your legs. Repeat 8-10 times.

3-Point Back Exercise

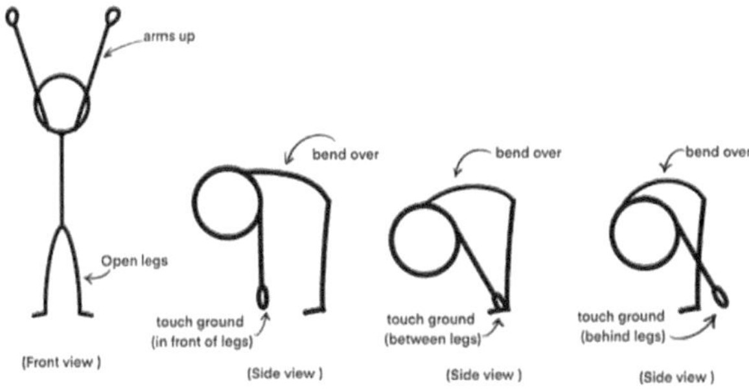

- **Sunlight**

  We need the sun on our bodies. I lay in sunlight 10-15 minutes a day, usually in the morning, before it gets too strong. Get as much body exposure as possible. Being naked is best.

- **Walking**

  Walking is great exercise. For some people, it's a lot healthier than running. I aim for 5,000-10,000 steps daily.

- **Vibration Plate Machine**

  5-10 minutes a day can help build bone density and relieve muscle soreness.

- **Infrared Sauna**

  20-25 mins (2-3 times a week) Great way to detox from our environment, which is full of toxins unfortunately.

- **Stretching**

  I stretch daily. There are a lot of stretches out there. Pick out the ones that work best for you.

- **Rolling**

  Use a muscle roller foam tube to roll your IT band. This can relieve knee and hip pain and avoid injuries.

- **Coffee Enemas**

  I do a coffee enema once a week to help cleanse the liver, which is your main organ for detoxing. It also helps me have regular bowel movements.

- **What To Eat**

  There is so much information and advice about eating it can make your head explode. But here are some simple guidelines to follow:

  Eat organic. Don't overeat. Eat for energy, not for comfort. Get a lot of color in your food. Before you put something you know is junk in your mouth, ask yourself, is it worth it?

  I eat mostly an ancestral food diet, based on Dr. Michael R. Rose's research, which is also known as paleo. It makes sense to me because it's what we were evolved to eat over hundreds of thousands of years before the advent of agriculture.

  I encourage you to pick a way of eating that works for you and stay on it.

2. HOLISTIC REGENERATIVE THERAPIES

- **PEMF Matt**

  Pulsed Electromagnetic Field mat supports healing and improved mobility by stimulating microcirculation, which we tend to lose as we age. I sleep on a mat set for that purpose, but just 10-20 minutes a day makes a real difference.

- **Ceragem Bed**

  This is a spinal massage bed that uses heat therapy to help your spine health. I've been doing it for years and use it about once a week.

- **Cold Plunge**

  I do a cold plunge that ranges from 40-50 degrees to boost my immunity and circulation and lower inflammation. You want to work up to sitting in it for three minutes, but give yourself time to get there. I do it once a week but would do more if I had one at home.

— OR —

- **Cryotherapy**

  Lowers your body temperature using liquid nitrogen, to reduce inflammation, and stimulate your immune system. This is an alternative to the cold plunge if it's more comfortable for you.

- **Colonics**

  Cleanses out your entire colon, which an enema won't do. I do these about twice a year. I did my first one when I was nine or ten.

- **Hydrogen Water**

  Regular water infused with H2, hydrogen water reduces inflammation and speeds up recovery time after workouts. It also can reduce fatigue and increase endurance. It's recommended to drink 2-3 glasses a day to be effective.

- **Hyperbaric Chamber**

  Hyperbaric oxygenates your blood stream, which can help with wound healing, killing pathogens and other benefits. I do five sessions twice a year.

- **Massage**

  Human touch is vital for longevity. Massage is a great way to release muscle tension and keep you moving right. I alternate between acupressure, deep tissue, and myofascial release. I try to get some form of massage every other week.

- **OsteoStrong**

  This is a great system for building bone density without injury. You can't do it at home. You have to go to them. I go there once a week to complete a 10–15-minute routine, using their unique machines, which has increased my bone density by 20%.

- **InfraRed light therapy**

  It's good for the skin and to heal wounds and get rid of soreness. I do this about three times week in total.

- **Super Patches Therapy**

  This is a new technology that works via your skin to optimize your neural network, without chemicals, for a range of benefits. I use patches to improve focus, sleep, strength, and flexibility.

- **Therapeutic Immune IVs**

When I feel a bug might be coming on, or I'm trying to get over something faster, I get an immune IV with glutathione, Vitamin C, and other good stuff.

3. ADVANCED PROTOCOLS

- **EBOO and EBOO2**

  Extracorporeal Blood Oxygenation and Ozonation (EBOO) takes 2 to 3 liters of your blood out in order to treat it with oxygen and ozone, then return it to your body. Takes about an hour to an hour and a half. It's a full body detoxification. I do it twice a year.

- **Therapeutic Plasma Exchange**

  This is a procedure that removes the plasma from your body, which may contain harmful antibodies or other disease-causing substances. This is another powerful detox treatment, which I do annually.

- **Whole Body Stem Cell Infusion**

  This infusion allows stem cells to travel throughout the bloodstream and to replace damaged cells and regenerate tissue. There are different kinds of stem cells and it's important to source them from quality suppliers. I use placenta stem cells, which are thought to be less likely to stimulate any latent cancer cells. I do this every other year.

- **Whole Body Exosome Infusion**

  Exosomes are the signaling molecules found in stem cells. But unlike stem cells, they are not living cells, and are considered safer because they lack DNA. I do this procedure annually to help rejuvenate skin and other organs and regenerate tissue where needed.

- **Peptides**

  I have used BPC-157 for healing tissue and anti-inflammatory effects, and Kisspeptin to support testosterone and libido. But there are many peptides becoming available for longevity and I am considering others.

CHAPTER 10

Travel Light: Seek and Ye Shall Find

". . . not my will, but thine, be done."

— Luke 22:42

* * * * *

"Don't carry yesterday with you."

— Luke 9:60–62

Now that you've read about my experience of the immortal lineage, you're ready to experience for yourself.

The Kingdom is here now. Jesus surrendered to this reality in his body. When he did that, he created a new lineage, an immortal lineage, that is separate from the lineage of struggle and sacrifice we were all born into. It wasn't his sacrifice and death that can save you. It was his passion for living and for people, which he imprinted into humankind. This is the gift he left all of us. This immortal lineage is your inheritance if you receive it.

We're conditioned to hearing limited answers to life's problems. We've tried many ways to feel happy, and even enlightened. But no matter what we try, it never seems to last. We might have moments of joy, but then the clouds close in. Because that is the way the program of mortality is designed. But this is different. This is a rebirth. You're reborn into the immortal lineage.

All we have to do, like Jesus did, is to surrender to what is already within us. This isn't another goal to set, or another New Years resolution you might struggle to fulfill. This immortal lineage is your inheritance. But we live in a noisy world full of distractions both inside and out. We do need to give our immortal lineage our faith. The more you focus with faith on this lineage the more vivid it will become.

You're going to almost want to pinch yourself. Because you're not yo-yoing any more between joy and sorrow. Because you're not running the program of survival anxiety anymore. You're finally getting to live who you really are.

Call Out to Your Lineage

You're going to start having such a deep feeling for your own person that you'll begin having communion with your own body. Instead of watching TV, you might want to just sit quietly and listen to your body. All your life, you've heard the sound of the system that is suppressing the body and ravaging the immune system and making life hard and unsustainable. You've been at war with yourself. Now you're opening to hear the sound of your body that has nothing but good news for you. The more you listen, the more you'll begin to recognize the difference.

Jesus said, call upon me and your burdens will be lifted. That's what you're doing. You're calling on your immortal body where he's imprinted in you. This is your real identity, the real you, not the program that enslaved you.

We've never really trusted our bodies a hundred percent. Your body is the Promised Land. Begin to listen to what your body is telling you. Ask for the will of your body to be done to transcend the program of death you've been made to serve. The mind is supposed to serve the body, not enslave it to fixed fears, dogmas, and limitations.

The more you listen for the voice of your immortal lineage, the more it will come forth. Jesus said seek and ye shall find, and you will. But the seeking isn't out in the world somewhere. It's not for a job, or a lover, or a product at the mall. The seeking is within, and with others who are taking the same journey into the Gospel of Longevity.

If you're driving to work, instead of getting frustrated with the traffic or worried about what's going to happen at your office, make this a divine time, a time for you. Consider it a blessing and use it to listen for your immortal lineage. That's the voice inside you that says let's move towards love, let's move toward light.

We don't realize this, but we've given our focus everywhere else except to the treasures that reside within us. Call on your body as you fall asleep at night that the will of your flesh will be done in the morning. Maybe it's a prayer, or a conversation with your bed partner. Or just a thought or a feeling that you're done with surviving. This is your time to enter into the Kingdom. And there's no struggle.

When you wake up in the morning, wake up with gratitude for being alive. Instead of listening to the voices of the negativity all around us, call forth the voice of this lineage. It's the voice you maybe only hear every once in a while, the voice that tells you beautiful things. But now you're opening to hear it all the time. You're letting yourself experience the divinity of your own person. This is the voice that is coming from the very core of your being. Go out in the sunlight and feel your body.

Don't worry about how fast or slow your transformation is going. Be patient with yourself. You're having a reborn experience and it's going to get greater and greater the more you give to it. But you're in charge. There are things you can do to accelerate your rebirth.

Talk About It with Others

The immortal lineage is a shared experience that is amplified in your body by talking about it with others. There's a reason why Jesus wandered in the wildness, but he didn't stay out there. He didn't find a cave to live in. He came back to his people. He wanted to talk to others. He wanted to connect, to share the experience.

Jesus said, *"For where two or three are gathered in my name, there am I in the midst of them."*—Matthew 18:20. What did he mean? He meant when we get together to open our experience of this lineage and to fellowship one another, our divinity becomes more present in our bodies, and we move each other to new places.

Seek out people you can have this conversation with. People Unlimited hold events every week dedicated to the Gospel of Longevity. You can join us online or in person. It's vital for you to have communion with others. Just go to www.peopleunlimitedinc.com.

Talk to the people in your life. Tell them about what's happening with you. Invite them to share in the experience. This lineage is in everyone. Some of us are just more aware of it than others.

Tell the people closest to you about the *Gospel of Longevity.* If they don't feel what you feel, don't struggle with them. Don't try to convince anyone of anything. Just share with them as much as you can. Be warm, be loving. But keep moving forward in your exploration of the Kingdom. Maybe they will come around. Your aliveness is contagious. Let the spirit of life that is in your body flow freely. Jesus said it only takes the faith the size of a mustard seed to trigger this rebirth. But even if they never come around, be at peace with them, and with everyone around you.

Don't fall into the trap of trying to fix people or yourself. You don't need fixing and neither does anyone else. You're not here to fix yourself, you're here to get in touch with who you really are.

You're already home in your own body. If you feel led to change a pattern in your life that isn't healthy for you, great. But don't make changing patterns your focus. Keep your eye on the life that you are. You'll see the negative patterns falling away. It may take effort, but it won't be a struggle.

Being in the Kingdom will change destructive patterns because your life is no longer about struggle. The more you feel the Gospel of Longevity, the more you're going to want to eat the right foods, and care for your body. You're going to feel much more satisfied with yourself, because you're finally living your body without all the judgements and agendas, that you're not going to need to try to medicate yourself with addictions of any kind.

Let Negativity Go

I used to be addicted to the news. I'd wake up in the morning and turn on the news. I would watch it and get so upset and I would just watch more. Which is exactly what these news shows want you to do. They want to hook you into what's wrong with the world. This response is programmed into us by evolution. Survival anxiety keeps us focused on what's wrong because the survival program sees that as the threat. This is also why insults tend to impact us more than compliments. Of course, this also consumes our spirit and makes longevity seem not only impossible but undesirable even if it was possible. Who wants to worry forever?

But since my reborn experience, I've lost my appetite for negativity. I don't watch a lot of news anymore and I'm not missing anything. I don't need to see every story about people doing worse than me to feel good about my life. I feel great about my life because I'm living my immortal lineage.

I'm not worried about the condition of the world. There's nothing new about the condition of the world—it's always been a world of struggle and strife, with sparks of beauty flashing here and there. But I'm not part of this world anymore. I've been born out of it. Doesn't mean I don't care. I do; I care deeply. I just know the solution won't come from inside the system that is wreaking this havoc in the first place. The best thing I can do for the world is to live my immortal lineage and spread the Gospel of Longevity. It's the only thing that makes peace on earth even possible.

Eat What Feeds Your Soul

Sometimes I find myself bored with empty entertainment. I want stuff that feeds my soul. Anytime I can watch or read something about Jesus, I do it. Granted, some of it is just religious propaganda that romanticizes his death and preaches doctrines that weren't even what he was about. But there is very moving material out there as well. Sometimes we have to look with new eyes at the old stories and find what is substantial and inspiring to us.

Some people feel anything from religion is tainted by the wrongs of the institutions that claim religious authority. Others are suspicious of science because it is too abstract for them to understand or contradicts some religious dogma. But when you're reborn, you lose the prejudice about where your inspiration has to come from. You open your body for what feeds you. You're no longer concerned with who would approve or disapprove, including your old self.

I go back and rewatch episodes of *The Chosen* that move me. I listen to gospel and spiritual music. I find stories from the Old Testament moving as well. I'm also inspired by the brilliant work of scientists working to cure aging, and by great people from history like Nelson Mandela and Abraham Lincoln. I don't need to be self-righteous about where the inspiration comes from. I just need to receive it.

Setbacks Aren't a Sin

Don't worry about setbacks, you're going to have them. You're making a huge move in your life. You're not always going to get it just right. Like in a football game, you might lose some yards down the field, but it doesn't really matter. You've got the next play and the next one and you're going to keep going.

We've been tied up in our bodies with trying to do everything right. We try to say the right things, and think the right thoughts, and the whole time feeling the pressure of survival pushing us in exactly the opposite direction. Now, we're taking the survival pressure off our bodies. We're letting go of that burden. Doing what's right for ourselves and others isn't a strain anymore.

Travel Light

We don't need nearly as much as we might think to live our immortal lineage. We can get weighed down with everything. When you have too many things and you're always wanting more, you're never satisfied and you never experience the fulfillment of your true inheritance.

People with power tend to want more power. People with wealth tend to want more wealth. Why is it never enough? Because they are still living in the system of sacrifice that is going to take everything in the end. I'm not serving that system anymore. I'm not trying to keep up with the Jones' or impress friend and family. I'm impressing the Lord, which is my body.

We need to travel light, financially and in every other way. That doesn't mean going without; it means going without the stresses that wear us out.

Recently, I was inspired to sell the building I'd owned for twenty years. People Unlimited met there, and my team worked in office space there as well. I was proud of that building and we had an impressive meeting space. In a way, it was a monument to our movement. But it was also a financial burden for me to carry. And I decided the only real monument to living is living. I recently closed the sale, and I feel much lighter, not because I'm retiring, but because I can focus more on spreading the Gospel of Longevity.

Debt is a big burden. I'm using some of the proceeds to pay off debt and I don't plan to take it on again. Debt is an American institution, but I'm living in the Kingdom now. I don't need all the stuff that people go into debt for. I'd rather feel the lightness of my spirit and be freed up to work on what really matters to me.

We're also planning on downsizing at home. We tend to collect a lot of stuff over time, and that stuff weighs us down. Then when you move, you realize how much of it you don't use at all. You don't have to wait to move house. Why not get rid of that old stuff sitting around right now? It will make your home more restful and your spirit lighter.

We hold on to so much in the way of experiences as well. We collect all sorts of history in our bodies, which weighs us down. Good things and bad, but especially the bad seems to accumulate and accumulate. It's like we're emotional hoarders. We're carrying too much to walk on water, and we sink. No wonder our longevity has been limited. We think eighty years is a long time because we carry all that baggage through those years. Think how much further we can go without carrying all those burdens of experience with us.

Traveling light might sound simple, and in many ways it is. But I truly believe this is the most powerful longevity body hack that's available today. This will build new resilience and joy for staying. It will allow your immune system to function better, because you aren't being drained by things that don't even matter anymore.

Don't struggle to unwind all the experiences that have marked you. I honestly don't believe it's possible anyway. The more we dig into what we feel is wrong with us, the more we find it. But when you open to your immortal lineage, the old seems to fall away. You start to feel the blessings that await you, instead of the curses that have troubled you. The traumas and frustrations that grow heavy in our bodies over time are aging to us. Now it's time to feel the freshness of life again.

The sheer vastness of the Kingdom raises you up and you realize there is a bigger life for you to live, which swallows up the struggles of the past in your body. You're beginning to glimpse the reality that we can have heaven here on earth. We stand at the end of the era of sacrifice and at the advent of the era of creation. There is no end to the goodness of this Kingdom and to our continual expansion within it. We are no longer waiting in disappointment and despair on the outside looking in. We are feeling the redemption of our bodies, and our hearts are filling with the joy and abundance of immortal human living.

Epilogue

Now that you've read my book, hopefully you understand that the time is now for us to live fully as never before. As Jesus said, the Kingdom is here now. And each of us is a mansion in this Kingdom.

Of course, not everyone is feeling this way. If only they were! So it's important to find like-minded people and spread the word to them so they can benefit too.

Like anything in life, the experience of being in the Kingdom is amplified when we share it with others. That's why I encourage you to share this book with the people you know and talk about your own experience of the Gospel of Longevity. You'll find that this creates a very special connection, a communion that expands our immortal spirit and energizes our aliveness.

This gospel is not a fixed doctrine. We are continuing to explore our Kingdom at my organization, People Unlimited, where we have weekly meetings. You can join in that conversation online or in person to keep feeding your spirit of aliveness. You can find out more at www.peopleunlimitedinc.com.

I'm on a mission to spread this Gospel of Longevity to every person who wants it. I would love to come to speak to your community, church, synagogue, mosque or temple. Please contact me at james@jamesstrole.com to discuss such opportunities.

And above all, I encourage you not to struggle with the system of survival that has held us all back. Instead, live your immortal inheritance to the fullest today and every day. Amen.

About the Authors

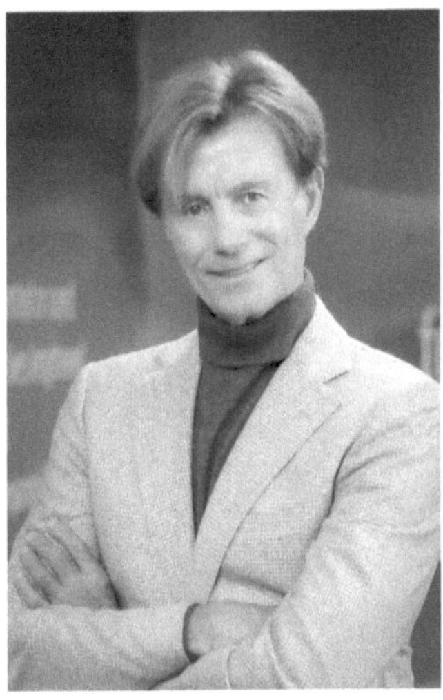

Photo credit - Augusto Herrera

JAMES R. STROLE

James Strole is a visionary futurist dedicated to helping bring about a world in which vibrant unlimited human lifespans are the norm. He is Executive Director of the not-for-profit Coalition for Radical Life Extension, which is the producer of RAADfest, the most comprehensive, science-based longevity event for a general audience. James is also the Director of People Unlimited, an international organization that supports people pursuing unlimited lifespans.

James has dedicated his life to challenging death-oriented beliefs and practices and has coached thousands of people in living an ageless lifestyle to achieve healthier, fuller, more satisfying lives. He has spoken and written on radical life extension and physical immortality for five decades. He has appeared on numerous TV shows both domestically and abroad and has spoken to audiences in twenty-six countries on four continents.

James is the creator of the *Gospel of Longevity*, an emotional and spiritual platform for immortal living. As James says: "We were all born into a mortal world and have operated from that mortal consciousness that rejects immortality. But there is also within us an immortal seed for us to tap into that calls us out of survival into a future of creativity and unlimited life."

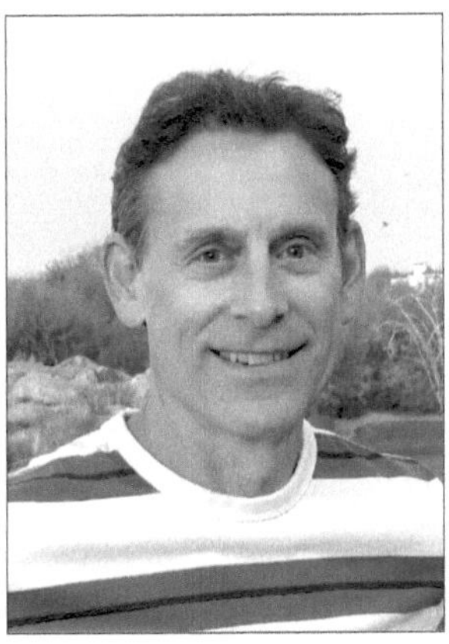

Photo credit - Leslie Calkins

JOSEPH BARDIN

Joe is a writer, speaker and strategist. He is the author of the essay collection *Outlier Heart* (IFERS Press). His essays have appeared in numerous publications including *Interim, Allium Journal, Louisville Review, Vol. 1 Brooklyn*, and *Eclectica*, among others, and been anthologized in the *Transhumanist Handbook* (Springer). His plays have been developed or produced in New York City, Chicago, Washington DC, San Diego, Tucson, Phoenix, and Kaiserslautern, Germany.

Joe is Director of Communications for the Coalition for Radical Life Extension and People Unlimited. As an activist for advancing transhumanism and immortalist thought, and democratizing access to longevity information and care, he has spoken throughout the US and internationally.

www.ingramcontent.com/pod-product-compliance
Ingram Content Group UK Ltd.
Pitfield, Milton Keynes, MK11 3LW, UK
UKHW041846200726
13854UKWH00005BA/2324

9 798885 812443